Guide to Federal Pharmacy Law

9th Edition

Barry S. Reiss, Ph.D.
Professor Emeritus
Albany College of Pharmacy
Albany, New York

Gary D. Hall, M.S.
Professor of Pharmaceutics
Albany College of Pharmacy
Albany, New York

Apothecary Press
Boynton Beach, FL

www.apothecarypress.com

ISBN 978-0-9676332-8-2

Printed in the United States of America

Preface

On behalf of Apothecary Press and the authors, we welcome you to our Guide to Federal Pharmacy Law, 9th Edition. This Guide has been prepared to assist you in making your review of federal pharmacy law as simple and painless as possible. As a comprehensive federal law review, we have become one of the most popular pharmacy law sources in the U.S. It has also become the most popular review manual for pharmacy students who are preparing for the MPJE® exam.

The Guide is divided into fourteen sections. Within some sections there are sample questions similar to the type that may be seen on the MPJE®. Answers to these questions are provided immediately following the questions. In this edition we have made some important additions, including changes in rescheduling of controlled substances, medical marijuana programs, FDA regulation of compounding, changes in Medicare, the Drug Quality and Securities Act (DQSA), and many other changes that have occurred since the last edition.

At the end of this Guide are 300 multiple-choice questions that cover the federal statutes, rules and regulations addressed by this book. Readers are encouraged to tackle these questions only after they have completed studying the contents of this Guide. This will serve as a practice examination that will help to identify areas of weakness that require further study. Answers to these questions may be found at the very end of the question section.

We thank the many pharmacy law faculty who have adopted our guide for their pharmacy law classes. We also thank the many pharmacy students who have contributed excellent critiques after having used our guide.

All the best,

Barry S. Reiss

Gary D. Hall

Contents

Section L

Section M

Section N

Section A

Guide to the MPJE®

Applying for and Taking the MPJE®

The MPJE® is a computerized law examination, which is required in most states for individuals to obtain a pharmacist license. Pharmacists attempting to reciprocate their licenses to another state are also often required to pass the MPJE®. The examination consists of questions based upon both federal drug laws and regulations and upon the laws and regulations of the specific state in which the exam is being taken.

All candidates are advised to obtain the latest copy of the NAPLEX®/MPJE® Registration Bulletin, which may be downloaded from NABP's website at

http://www.nabp.net/programs/examination/mpje/registration-bulletin

This bulletin is updated on a regular basis and describes the procedures for applying for and taking the computerized examination.

Remember that each state has established its own criteria for determining a candidate's eligibility to take the MPJE® examination. However, the following guidelines may be useful to simplify the application process:

- Carefully review the NABP®'s Registration Bulletin because changes may be made to the guidelines at any time.
- Complete the registration form and mail it to your STATE BOARD OF PHARMACY with the required fees. Be sure to apply for the appropriate licensing examination (i.e. either the NAPLEX® or the MPJE®).
- Your state's board of pharmacy will notify NABP® of your eli-

gibility to take the licensing examination.

- If you are qualified to take an examination, an Authorization to Test (ATT) will be sent to you. It will indicate the dates of your eligibility, an ATT number, a candidate identification number, and an expiration date (usually about one year).
- You may contact any testing center location to schedule your individual testing time. Presently, Pearson VUE testing centers are being used. When contacting the testing site, have the following available:
  - — Authorization number
  - — Candidate ID number
  - — Expiration date from your ATT card
- Arrive at the testing center at least 15 minutes early. Have available:
  - — Your ATT.
  - — Two forms of identification, at least one of which must have a picture ID with signature. (Driver's license or passport is acceptable).
- The computerized examination must be completed in two hours. Extra time will be provided to complete a questionnaire and a short tutorial.
- No food, drink, reference books, or notes are allowed.
- You are not permitted to open personal belongings such as bags or wallets during the exam.
- Your examination score will be reported only to the board of pharmacy of the state you have designated.

Content of the MPJE®

As of September 1, 2016 the MPJE® examination will consist of 90 multiple-choice questions of which 75 will contribute to your score. The remaining 15 are intermingled throughout the exam and are "pretest questions" that do not count toward your score. That is, they are new questions, which the NABP is evaluating for level of difficulty and appropriateness. Some of these may show up in later examinations as questions that will count!

The level of difficulty for MPJE® questions will vary. While the passing score for the exam is set at 75, it does NOT mean that you have to correctly answer at least 75% of the questions in order to pass. The actual number of correct answers needed to pass a specific examination may vary from one exam to another.

The person next to you may have some test questions that are different from yours in wording, topics covered, and degree of difficulty. The cardinal rule to remember is simply to answer ALL questions to the best of your ability. Do not become discouraged if you have several very difficult questions.

As of March 1, 2013 candidates are permitted five attempts to pass the MPJE® examination for each jurisdiction or state. An additional attempt may be granted by the board of pharmacy.

The examination will have questions involving federal laws and regulations as well as specific state laws and regulations. The questions will be intermingled. Clearly, you should be familiar with not only the federal laws and regulations, but also those of the state to which you are applying. Because each state has its own unique laws, this Guide is focused only on federal laws and regulations

MPJE® Competency Statements

As of April, 2016, the NABP® has established a set of competency statements, which serve as a blueprint of the topics covered on the exam. The MPJE® Bulletin describes the three major areas included in the examination. These consist of:

Area 1	Pharmacy Practice (approximately 83% of exam)
Area 2	Licensure, Registration, Certification, and Operational Requirements (approximately 15% of exam)
Area 3	General Regulatory Processes (approximately 2% of exam)

The candidate may wish to review the competencies listed under each of the above areas. However, the statements are not very descriptive. Obviously the examination will stress those laws and regulations with which any individual entering the profession should be familiar. These will include:

- Requirements for obtaining and maintaining a pharmacist license including continuing education requirements.
- The structure and duties of a board of pharmacy and authorized inspection bodies.
- The standards of practice for both the filling and refilling of prescriptions.
- State drug substitution requirements.
- Procedures for the purchase, storage, and record keeping of drugs.
- Regulations for counseling of patients and guaranteeing the confidentiality of their prescriptions and medical records.
- Requirements for the registration and maintenance of a pharmacy whether in a community or institutional setting.
- Additional requirements for the purchase, storage, record keeping, and dispensing of controlled substances.
- The pathways and requirements for bringing new drugs to the market.

- Individual laws and regulations, of either state or federal origin, which impact upon the practice of pharmacy (e.g. Orphan Drug Act).

While some of the above concepts are described in individual state law, many are under the jurisdiction of federal agencies; for example, the labeling of OTC's (nonprescription drugs), dietary and nutritional supplements, and cosmetics.

Remember that almost all rules and regulations involving hospitals, nursing homes, and other health-related organizations located within a given state are promulgated by that individual state, not the federal government.

Study Tip

Obviously you must review both the federal and your specific state's pharmacy laws since approximately 50% of your exam will be based upon state law. This review book is intended to concentrate on federal pharmacy law, which is appropriate for all states.

It is the objective of this book to review material most likely to be on your exam. Naturally there will always be a few questions from "left field" that were neither presented in this Guide or in your pharmacy college's Jurisprudence course.

Don't worry about the isolated facts. Instead, concentrate on major topics. You are fortunate if you are taking the exam in a state that closely follows federal law.

Study Tip

In reviewing for the exam, your objective is to learn the law and to recognize what areas of the law are applicable in a particular question. DO NOT attempt to memorize the exact citation for a law such as 503; 21 U.S.C. 353 for the Durham-Humphrey Amendment or a state regulation designation such as "Section 2857" of the Public Health Law. While it may be useful to learn the date of origin for major laws such as the FD&C Act of 1938, it is very unlikely that you will be questioned on the dates of less significant legislation.

Remember also that when legislation is passed, it may not immediately take effect. For example, The Durham-Humphrey Amendment was passed by Congress in 1951 but did not become effective until 1952.

Spend most of your review time on questions related to the federal Controlled Substances Act. Obviously it is also important to concentrate on your individual state's pharmacy laws and regulations.

When reviewing specific laws and regulations, carefully note the difference between the designations of "shall" and "may". The term "shall" like the term "must" is an absolute requirement. The term "may" is looser, indicating the permission to do something. For example, "the pharmacist shall place poison prevention closures on prescription containers" versus "the pharmacist may supply prescription package inserts to a patient when dispensing a drug".

Questions on the MPJE® are likely to be in one of two formats. Many questions will have a simple stem followed by five choices lettered A through E. The candidate must select the BEST answer and key that answer into the computer. Other questions will be in the format known as multi-response questions, combined response, or "K" questions. These simply refer to questions with a simple stem followed by three choices numbered I, II, and III. The answer choices will consist of several single and combinations of these three choices. The format always used for answer choices in "K" questions is:

(A) I only

(B) III only

(C) I and II only

(D) II and III only

(E) I, II, and III

"K" questions are frequently found on the NAPLEX® and, to a lesser extent, on the MPJE®. These questions are usually considered to be more difficult than standard multiple-choice questions since the candidate is not just seeking a single correct answer but possible combinations of correct answers. While many federal laws and regulations are complex, MPJE® examiners are generally realistic and are unlikely to ask the candidate to identify obscure facts about federal laws.

Study Tip

When answering a "K" question, ignore the combinations of answers until you have closely evaluated each choice. For each, decide if it is true or correct, and then hope that your answer is among the choices offered. For example, if you decide that I and II are correct answers and III is not, obviously you would key in (C) as the answer. However if you have selected the combination of I and III, you will quickly notice that this combination is not a selection in the answer key. Obviously you should reconsider as to whether just I or III are correct or if it is possible that II is also correct?

A second situation occurs when you have decided that III is correct, I is not correct, but you are uncertain about choice II. It is probably better to go with what you know to be correct, i.e., the choice of III only.

Other things to remember while you are taking the MPJE® include:

- Read each question carefully and try to determine what concept, general principle or specific law is being tested. Remember that when there is a conflict between federal and an individual state's law, the stricter law usually applies (e.g. if a controlled drug is federally classified in Schedule III and is classified by the state as a Schedule II drug, the more stringent state law applies).
- When a question mentions a specific drug, try to classify it in your mind as a controlled substance, non-controlled prescription-only drug or OTC.
- Assume that each question has been written in a straightforward manner. The examiners are not out to trick you.

- After deciding upon the correct response, complete the answering process using three steps.
  1. Highlight the answer on the computer screen.
  2. Request the next question by keying the icon on the lower right portion of the screen.
  3. Confirm that you want the next question by keying the icon next to the above icon.

> ### Note
>
> Remember that once you have completed steps 2 and 3, you are NOT permitted to return to the previous question and change your answer. Don't hurry through questions and risk a quick decision. You have plenty of time to complete the examination. On the other hand, don't over analyze the questions. Your first choice is probably the best choice.

Scoring of your MPJE® is done very quickly and the results are sent to the board(s) of pharmacy you have designated. Remember that you have no way of knowing how well you are doing during the exam. Do not become discouraged if you run into several difficult questions. Simply answer ALL questions to the best of your ability and knowledge. While the passing grade is set at 75%, this does not mean that you have to correctly answer a minimum of 75% of the questions. It is possible that a raw score of below 75% will convert into a passing grade.

Common Errors Made By Candidates

- ***Not reading the question carefully***

  Example: Which one of the following is NOT required to be placed by the pharmacist onto a prescription?

  vs.

  Which one of the following is NOT required to be placed by the pharmacist onto a prescription label?

- ***Basing your answers on your knowledge of local laws or regulations.***

  Example: Expiration dating on prescription labels is NOT required by either federal or most state laws but may be a state or local requirement.

- ***Basing your answers on what you do in the pharmacy you are employed in.***

  Unfortunately, some pharmacies do not follow the letter of the law. Using your pharmacy's current practice as a guideline for choosing your answer may result in incorrect answers on this examination.

- ***Attempting to base an answer on recent changes in the law.***

  New laws or regulations may be ambiguous or poorly understood by practitioners. For this reason, questions on the MPJE® exam are usually based on well-established laws and regulations. If a question is based on a fairly recent law, it is likely to be a question that is being tested by NABP® and will likely not count toward the calculation of your score.

Section B

Sources of Laws, Rules and Regulations

Introduction

Many laws and amendments that have shaped the current Food, Drug and Cosmetic Act were enacted over the past 100 years. In most cases they represent attempts on the part of lawmakers to protect the American public.

Pure Food and Drug Act of 1906

Up to 1906 there were relatively few controls on the distribution of foods, drug-containing products, cosmetic products and medical devices. Products were often contaminated, were not consistent in strength and were poorly labeled. In 1906 Congress passed the Pure Food and Drug Act. This law prohibited foods and drugs that were distributed through interstate commerce to be adulterated or misbranded. The law fell short of protecting the public since it did not require manufacturers to list on the label the ingredients or directions for use of a product. The law also did not regulate cosmetic products or medical devices.

Food, Drug and Cosmetic Act of 1938

In 1937, 107 deaths caused by the mistaken use of diethylene glycol (automobile anti-freeze), as a vehicle in a sulfanilamide elixir resulted in the passage of a landmark piece of federal regulation, the Food, Drug and Cosmetic Act (FDCA) of 1938. This law required, for the first time in the US, that any new drug could not be marketed unless it had first been proven to be safe when used according to directions on the label. It also required that labels include adequate directions for use and warnings about habit-forming drugs that were contained in the product. It was also the first law that applied to cosmetic products and medical devices as well as to food and drug products.

Drug products marketed prior to 1938 were exempted or "grandfathered" and did not, therefore, have to be labeled or proven safe under this law. The FDCA became the backbone of many subsequent laws and amendments that further strengthened drug control in the US.

> ***Note***
>
> Several drug products still sold in pharmacies (e.g. levothyroxine, digoxin, nitroglycerin, and phenobarbital) were on the market prior to 1938 and are, therefore, still "grandfathered" from this law.

Durham-Humphrey Amendment of 1951

Many of the drug products covered by the 1938 FDCA Act were not safe to use without medical supervision. The Durham-Humphrey Amendment of 1951 was enacted to further regulate these products. This was an amendment to the FDCA that established two classes of drugs. Those that required medical supervision to be used safely did not have to list "adequate directions for use" but were required to include the legend "Caution: Federal law prohibits dispensing without a prescription" on the manufacturer's label.

The requirement for "adequate directions for use" was satisfied by the pharmacist placing directions provided by the prescriber on the label of the dispensed product (e.g. Take one tablet twice daily). Such products became known as prescription or "legend" drugs.

Products that did not require medical supervision for their use had to have adequate directions for use on their label and were referred to as "over-the-counter" (OTC) or nonprescription drug products. In addition to distinguishing between legend and nonprescription drug products, this legislation also provided for oral prescriptions and prescription refills.

Kefauver-Harris Amendment of 1962

The Kefauver-Harris Amendment was adopted as a result of public concern about thalidomide, a sedative-hypnotic drug. This drug was marketed in Europe but was not approved by the FDA for the US market. In 1961, it was determined that thalidomide had caused serious birth defects in the offspring of many women in Europe who had used the drug.

While there were few birth defects seen in the US, Congress enacted the Kefauver-Harris Amendment to protect the public in the future. This amendment to the FDCA Act (also referred to as the Drug Efficacy Amendment) required that all new drugs marketed in the US had to be shown to be not only safe, but also effective. This requirement was also extended to products that had been approved between 1938 and 1962.

In addition to this efficacy requirement, the Amendment also included provisions that placed the authority for regulating prescription drug advertising into the hands of the FDA. It also required informed consent for individuals who were research subjects in clinical investigations, reporting of adverse drug reactions, and creation of Good Manufacturing Practice (GMP) requirements that clearly defined the conditions under which drugs could be manufactured in the US.

Study Tip

Remember that prescription drug advertising is regulated by the FDA. Nonprescription (OTC) advertising is regulated by the Federal Trade Commission (FTC).

Medical Device Amendment of 1976

In order to protect the American public against potentially dangerous or useless medical devices, Congress enacted the Medical Device Amendment of 1976. This amendment to the FDCA Act provides for better classification of medical devices according to their specific function, establishment of performance standards for these devices, pre-market approval requirements, conformance with GMP standards, and requirements for adherence to record and reporting requirements.

Orphan Drug Act of 1983

Orphan drugs are those that are used to treat diseases that are relatively rare, i.e. they affect relatively few people. Prior to 1983 the cost of developing and marketing such drugs was prohibitive for most drug manufacturers because of their limited potential for profitability. In 1983, Congress enacted the Orphan Drug Act. This provided various tax and licensing incentives to manufacturers, thereby making development of such drugs more appealing. A rare disease is usually considered one that affects less than 200,000 persons in the United States.

Drug Price Competition and Patent-Term Restoration Act

This piece of legislation, sometimes called the Hatch-Waxman Amendment, attempted to resolve a dispute between generic drug and brand name drug manufacturers. Prior to the enactment of this amendment to the FDCA, generic drug manufacturers had to go through most of the lengthy drug approval process that was required of manufacturers of newly developed drugs. New drug manufacturers were concerned about limited periods of exclusive patent rights for their innovative products.

In enacting this bill, Congress streamlined the drug approval process for generic products by requiring submission of only an abbreviated new drug application (ANDA). This generally does not require costly clinical testing for approval of a generic product. It only requires proof of bioequivalence with its brand-name counterpart. Brand name drug manufacturers were provided with incentives to develop new drug products by being awarded up to five additional years of patent protection to compensate them for the lengthy time it takes to go through the FDA approval process.

Prescription Drug Marketing Act of 1987

This bill was enacted in order to place more stringent controls on the distribution of prescription drug products and samples. Elements of this legislation include:

- Requiring that prescription drug wholesalers be licensed by states under federal guidelines.
- Banning re-importation of prescription drugs produced in the United States.
- Banning the sale, trade or purchase of prescription drug samples.
- Specifying precise storage, handling and recordkeeping requirements for drug samples.
- Prohibiting, with certain exceptions, the resale of prescription drugs purchased by hospitals or health care facilities.

FDA Modernization Act of 1997

This Act is a far-reaching piece of legislation that touches virtually every aspect of FDA's activities. Included in this legislation are the following:

- Provisions for the fast-track review of some New Drug Application submissions. The intent is to expedite the approval of new drugs used to treat serious or life-threatening conditions.

- Clarification of the conditions under which pharmacies may perform extemporaneous compounding of prescriptions. One premise is that individual states should regulate compounding. Also, pharmacies are exempt from the strict regulatory federal GMP standards and the requirements for submission of new drug applications.
- The prescription drug legend "Caution: Federal law prohibits dispensing without a prescription" is replaced by "Rx only".
- The provision that required certain substances to be labeled "Warning – May be habit forming." has been eliminated.
- Encouragement for manufacturers to conduct research for new uses of drugs and to submit supplemental NDAs for these uses. The manufacturers may publicly disseminate limited information about these unapproved uses provided a statement is included specifying that the use has not been approved or cleared by the FDA.
- Encouragement for drug manufacturers to perform pediatric studies of drugs by providing them with an additional six months of marketing exclusivity.

Medicare Prescription Drug Improvement, and Modernization Act of 2003

See Section D for a detailed discussion of this Act.

Patient Protection and Affordable Care Act (Health Care Reform Act) of 2010

After contentious debate, Congress passed a major bill in 2010 that affects health care delivery to all Americans. While portions of the provisions will go into effect almost immediately, others will be phased into place over several years. Questions concerning specifics of the Act are unlikely to be included on the MPJE®, especially since many provisions are likely to be clarified and/or changed over the next few years.

Among the areas of this legislation that affect pharmacist interactions with consumers, government agencies, and other health professionals include:

1. Require that all individuals have health insurance. A Health Insurance Exchange was created allowing individuals and families to purchase health coverage with credits available based upon their Federal Poverty Level (FPL). Small businesses also receive credits if they provide employee health coverage.
2. Require standards for financial and administrative transactions including timely and transparent claims using standard electronic transactions. (Previously enacted legislation required Part D pharmacy claims to be paid within 14 days after electronic submission or within 30 days if submitted by other means.)
3. Stop agreements between brand name and generic drug manufacturers that limit or delay competition from generic drugs.
4. Phase elimination of the catastrophic threshold, better known as the "donut hole" or "coverage gap", during which the patient pays all costs of prescription drugs.

Time lines for implementation of the Patient Protection and Affordable Care Act of 2010:

The passage of this law in 2010 established a time line for its implementation. The following is a summary of this time line.

2010

- Insurance companies are no longer allowed to deny coverage to children with pre-existing illnesses.

- Children are able to stay on their parent's health insurance policies until they turn 26 years old, i.e. through the age of 25.
- Individuals who have not had health insurance for six months receive a subsidy to enroll in high-risk insurance pools run by the states.
- All new insurance plans sold must exempt preventative care and screenings from deductibles.
- Small businesses with fewer than 25 employees receive up to a 35 percent tax credit for providing health insurance to their employees.

2011

- Senior citizens that fall into the "medicare donut hole" (a coverage gap) receive a 50% discount on some drugs.
- Employers also start to include the cost of health care on employee's W-2 forms.

2012

- The US Department of Health and Human Services (HHS) initiates the preparation of meaningful requirements for increasing the use of electronic health records (EHRs) and sets goals for 2013 and 2014. Stage 1 of this process establishes basic methods to enable electronic capture of patient data and provides electronic copies of health information to patients. Stage 2 extends beyond simple data capture to sharing of information between providers. It also promotes the patient's ability to access their health information. Stage 3 focuses on improving health outcomes through greater use of clinical decision support, increases patient engagement, and widens sharing of clinical data.

In 2012, **The Women's Preventive Health Care Amendment**, part of the Affordable Health Care Act, began providing services to women including

- well woman visits
- gestational diabetes screening
- Human papillomavirus screening
- STD counseling
- HIV counseling and screening
- contraceptive counseling
- etc.

These services are provided periodically without patient cost sharing.

2013

- Many of the new taxes and fees that pay for the health care bill become effective.

These taxes include new Medicare taxes on individuals who earn more than $200,000 a year. The wage tax, dividends and interest tax, and a small tax on medical devices are also implemented.

2014

- Exchanges are created so individuals without employer-provided health care (e.g. employees of small businesses) can shop for health care coverage
- Insurance companies are barred from denying coverage on the basis of pre-existing conditions.
- The insurance industry is required to pay an annual fee to help pay for the exchanges that cover all citizens that cannot otherwise receive insurance.

- In addition to providing subsidies and guaranteed coverage for most citizens, the new health care bill requires that most people have health insurance. There is a fine for not carrying some health insurance .
- An independent Medicare board is created to help curb Medicare costs if the costs rise more quickly than inflation.

2015

- The new health care bill continues the new coverage, taxes and fees that were created in previous years.

2016

- The penalty for individuals who do not purchase health insurance rises to a minimum of $695.

2017

- Businesses that have more than 100 employees would be allowed to participate in the state insurance exchanges, if the state government allows it.

2018

- An excise tax would be imposed on so-called "Cadillac plans" that generally provide more than $27,500 worth of coverage for a family.

CAUTION! Any of the provisions outlined in this section may be changed by either Congress or the HHS at any time. Thus, it is unlikely that the MPJE® will include detailed questions on the provisions.

Official Compendia of the United States

- ***United States Pharmacopoeia/National Formulary (USP/NF)***

  The US government does NOT publish this reference. It is published by a private organization known as the US Pharmacopoeia Convention (USPC). The *USP/NF* contains monographs of recognized drugs. Each monograph includes the drug's chemical characteristics and standards of quality. Proposed changes of the *USP/NF* are published in the *Pharmacopoeial Forum (PF)*, a bimonthly publication available in print and online. While printed as one bound book, the *USP* and *NF* are still considered to be two separate entities.

- ***Homeopathic Pharmacopoeia of the United States (HPUS)***

  This is also published by a private organization or convention that updates information about homeopathic products or remedies on a regular basis.

> **Note**
>
> If a drug is listed by its official name in the *USP/NF* or *HPUS*, it must meet the requirements specified in either book. Otherwise, it must have the designation "not *USP/NF*". Without this designation the drug is considered to be either misbranded or adulterated. If a drug is official in both the *USP/NF* and *HPUS*, it must meet the standards established in the *USP/NF* monograph unless it is distinctly marketed and labeled as a homeopathic drug.

Drugs@FDA

One of the most useful drug information resources is a website produced by the FDA, Center for Drug Evaluation and Research, known as Drugs@FDA. This is a searchable website that contains information about approved and tentatively approved prescription, nonprescription, and discontinued drugs. It also includes links to drug approval letters, labels, and scientific reviews. The primary uses of Drugs@FDA are to:

- find labels for approved drug products.
- find generic drug products for a brand name product.
- find all drug products with a specific active ingredient.
- view the regulatory history of an approved drug.
- find consumer information for drugs approved after 1998.
- find therapeutic equivalent drug products for a brand name or generic drug product.

Most of the information on this site can easily be downloaded into a spreadsheet format.

Section C

Acronyms and Definitions

The pharmacist is expected to have a working knowledge of health care terminology. It is, therefore, frustrating when one encounters an unfamiliar abbreviation or acronym. Throughout this Guide, we will use such abbreviations or acronyms. The following table will identify those most popularly used:

> ### *Study Tip*
>
> Fortunately, the MPJE® is a multiple-choice exam. It is, therefore, unlikely that you will be asked to identify the name of the organization with the acronym "CMS". However, a question could be worded: "What federal organization is responsible for administering Medicare?" Another question might be "Which federal department is responsible for the DEA?" (Ans.- The Department of Justice). It is probably sufficient if you review the following list and simply be able to recognize the meaning of these common acronyms.

Acronyms

AAC - Actual Acquisition Cost - the actual price a pharmacist pays when purchasing units of a drug product. This price usually represents a discounted price from the Average Wholesale Price (AWP).

AARP - American Association of Retired Persons

ADE or **ADR** - Adverse Drug Experience or Adverse Drug Reaction

AMP - Average Manufacturer Price – average price paid by wholesalers to a manufacturer for drugs that are to be sold at retail

ANDA - Abbreviated New Drug Application

ATF - Alcohol, Tobacco, and Firearms agency

AWP - Average Wholesale Price – a published wholesale price for a drug product that can be used as the basis for pricing prescription drugs. Usually pharmacies are able to purchase the drug at lower (discounted) prices from the AWP.

CAM – Complementary and Alternative Medicine

CDC - Centers for Disease Control

CDER - Center for Drug Evaluation and Research

CFR - Code of Federal Regulations – a compilation of final regulations and notices promulgated by the federal government; published annually by the US Government Printing Office; the above regulations and notices are first published in the *Federal Register*, a daily publication.

CMS - Centers for Medicare and Medicaid Services - responsible for administering Medicare and overseeing states' administration of Medicaid; formerly known as the Health Care Financing Administration

CPSC - Consumer Product Safety Commission

CSOS - Controlled Substance Ordering System - electronic substitute for DEA Form 222 when ordering Schedule I and/or II substances.

DEA - Drug Enforcement Administration - administration responsible for the federal Controlled Substances Act (CSA). It is part of the U.S. Department of Justice.

DHHS - Department of Health and Human Services - department which includes the Food and Drug Administration (FDA).

DI - Dietary Ingredient - may be a vitamin, mineral, herb or other botanical, an amino acid, or another dietary substance that supplements the diet.

DME - Durable Medical Equipment – equipment that meets three standards:

1. It can stand repeated use.
2. It is primarily for a medical purpose (i.e., it is not useful to a person if they have no illness or injury).
3. It is appropriate for use in the home. Examples of DME's include wheelchairs, oxygen tanks, and walkers.

DQSA - Drug Quality and Security Act

DRG's - Diagnosis Related Groups - a classification system for hospital inpatients based on the principal diagnosis; reimbursement is usually based on days of stay.

DS - Dietary Supplement - an over-the-counter product, containing one or more dietary ingredients, that is taken to improve upon a health condition, or simply enhance health, well being (mental and physical), or perhaps cosmetically to improve appearance.

DSHEA - Dietary Supplement Health Education Act

DUR - Drug Utilization Review – a review of prescription drug use, prescribing patterns or drug utilization by patients. Its purpose is to determine if appropriate drugs are being prescribed and if those drugs are being used appropriately.

EAC - Estimated Acquisition Cost – an estimated cost of a drug to a pharmacy based upon information collected by the DHHS (Department of Health and Human Services). Such costs are often based upon the quantity purchased.

EHR - Electronic Health Records - HHS requirements to encourage health professionals to share clinical information.

EOB - Electronic Orange Book

FDA - Food and Drug Administration

FDCA - Food, Drug and Cosmetic Act (FD & C Act or FDCA)

FTC - Federal Trade Commission – responsible for investigating unfair business practices including misleading advertising, etc.

GMP - Good Manufacturing Practice

GRAS - Generally Recognized As Safe – refers to a large number of relatively inert ingredients that are permitted to be used in pharmaceutical and food products as excipients or adjuvants because of their relatively high degree of safety.

GRASE - Generally Recognized as Safe and Effective - Term usually used when considering the safety and effectiveness of non-prescription product ingredients.

HCFA - Health Care Financing Administration – formerly responsible for policies relating to Medicare (federally managed) and Medicaid (controlled by individual states under the supervision of HCFA). Now referred to as Centers for Medicare and Medicaid Services (CMS).

HHA - Home Health Agency – an organization licensed or certified by the government to provide home health care services.

HIPAA - Health Insurance Portability and Accountability Act

HMO - Health Maintenance Organization

HP/HPUS - *Homeopathic Pharmacopoeia of the United States*

HSA - Health Savings Account

HSD - Home-use Sterile Drug products

IND - Investigational New Drug

JCAHO - Joint Commission on Accreditation of Health Care Organizations

LVP – Large Volume Parenteral

MAC - Maximum Allowable Cost – the highest price allowed under a specific plan for a specific drug (usually multi-source drugs). If a person wants a more expensive version, he/she must pay the difference.

NABP - National Association of Boards of Pharmacy (creates the NAPLEX® and MPJE®).

NDA – New Drug Application

NDC - National Drug Code – a classification system for identifying a specific drug product; used nationally for reimbursement and for identification of drug products.

NIH - National Institutes of Health

NDI - New Dietary Ingredient. Any substance that was not marketed as a dietary supplement ingredient in the U.S. prior to October 15, 1994. A manufacturer intending to market a New Dietary Ingredient must submit to the FDA, at least 75 days before introduction of the product into commerce, documented evidence establishing that the NDI is reasonably expected to be safe as used in the dietary supplement.

Non-DI - An excipient or other substance used in the manufacture of a dietary supplement (DS).

NPI - National Provider Identifier

OBRA - Omnibus Budget Reconciliation Act - act passed each year by Congress to fund many activities; each OBRA is known by the year it was enacted.

OSHA - Occupational Safety and Health Administration - responsible for monitoring the work environment to assure worker safety.

OTC - Over-the-Counter - refers to drugs and drug products, which are available without a prescription; also referred to as "non-prescription".

PBM - Pharmacy Benefits Management - organization that manages pharmaceutical benefits for managed care organizations or employers.

PFFS - Private fee-for-service plans that allow you to go to any doctor or hospital that accepts their terms.

PHS - Public Health Service

PI - Package Insert

PPI - Patient Package Insert

PPO - Preferred Provider Organization – a group of health professionals who are contractually favored to provide health services to individuals under a specific insurance plan.

PPPA - Poison Prevention Packaging Act

REMS - Risk Evaluation and Mitigation Strategy - FDA requirement for drug manufacturers to develop strategies to assure safe use of a specific drug.

SDA - Specially Denatured Alcohol

SNDA - Supplemental New Drug Application

SNF - Skilled Nursing Facility - a site that treats patients especially in need of rehabilitation or a lower level of medical care than is needed in a hospital.

SNP - Special Needs Plan - a category of Medicare Advantage plan designed for people living in long-term care facilities and receiving both Medicaid and Medicare or who have certain disabling chronic illnesses.

SP - Sterile Product or Supervising Pharmacist

TCAM - Traditional, complementary, and alternative medicine

TRP - Tamper Resistant Packaging

USAN - United States Adopted Names

USP/NF - *United States Pharmacopoeia/National Formulary*

USP DI - *United States Pharmacopoeia Dispensing Information* - a set of three volumes containing a variety of information, including:

- *Volume I - Drug Information for the Health Care Professional* - contains information about individual drugs. It is written specifically for health professionals.
- *Volume II - Advice for the Patient* – contains drug information in lay language and includes information intended for the general public about the use of drugs (side effects, etc.) Individual pages may be photocopied and provided to patients as part of the counseling process.
- *Volume III - Approved Drug Products With Therapeutic Equivalence Evaluations* - contains information from The Orange Book, *USP/NF* definitions and regulations, portions of the Federal Controlled Substances Act, plus other information.

VIPPS - Verified Internet Pharmacy Practice Site - List of relatively safe online pharmacies.

Definitions

Cosmetic - Article intended to be rubbed, poured, sprinkled, sprayed on, introduced into or otherwise applied to the human body for the purpose of cleansing, beautifying, promoting attractiveness, or altering the appearance. Also, any component of the above articles is considered to be a cosmetic.

> **Note**
>
> There is one exception to the above – Soap is not considered to be a cosmetic.

Device - Any instrument, apparatus, implement, machine, contrivance, implant, in vitro reagent or related article which is

- recognized in the *USP/NF* or *HPUS* or any supplement.
- intended for use in the diagnosis, cure, mitigation, treatment, or prevention of disease in man or other animals.
- intended to affect the structure or any function of the body of humans or animals but are not foods.

> **Note**
>
> Examples of devices would include infusion pumps, cardiac pacemakers and heart monitors.

Drug – Any of the following:

- Article recognized in the official *United States Pharmacopoeia/ National Formulary (USP/NF)*, or official *Homeopathic Pharmacopoeia of the United States (HPUS)*, or any supplements of these references.
- Article intended for use in the diagnosis, cure, mitigation, treatment, or prevention of disease in man or other animals.
- Article (other than food) intended to affect the structure or any function of the body of man or other animals.
- Article intended for use as a component of any articles specified in the above but does not include devices or their components, parts, or accessories.

Drug Sample - A unit of drug product not intended to be sold. Usually it is intended to acquaint a prescriber with a drug product by providing several doses for short-term or initial therapy.

Food - An article used for food or drink in humans or animals, chewing gum, and substances used as components of food or drink.

Note

It is unlikely that questions concerning subtle distinctions between foods, drugs, and cosmetics will be asked since there have been too many court decisions and changing opinions that cloud these distinctions. For example, minor claims for "anti-aging" creams have been accepted for cosmetic status while other creams containing hormones are considered to be drug products. Also, some chemicals with therapeutic uses have been classified as dietary supplements.

Generic Name - A name that is assigned to a specific drug structure. It is a simplified name as compared to the chemical name. Drug products may be marketed under their "generic name" or a brand name (trade name). The general perception is that a drug marketed under its generic name is usually less expensive than the brand name product.

Hospice - A facility or program that provides palliative and supportive care for terminally ill patients.

Sample Questions

1. Which one of the following acronyms does NOT refer to pharmacy economics?

   (A) AAC (B) ATF (C) AMP (D) EAC (E) MAC

2. Which one of the following acronyms directly relates to Alcohol?

   (A) AMP (B) ADE (C) CAM (D) GRAS (E) SDA

3. A list of safe online pharmacies will be found in which of the following sites?

   (A) HPUS (B) JCAHO (C) USAN (D) VIP (E) VIPPS

4. Hospital heath care reimbursement is most closely associated with which one of the following acronyms?

   (A) DRG (B) DEA (C) GMP

Answers:

(1) B (2) E (3) E (4) A

Section D

Medicare and Medicaid

The two major public medical reimbursement programs in the United States are Medicare and Medicaid. This book will focus primarily on Medicare laws and regulations since these are controlled by the federal government. While Medicaid payments are at least partially reimbursed by the federal government, the program is regulated by the individual states and coverage may vary from one state to another. Medicaid patients who move from one state to another must reapply for coverage and may encounter different requirements. In preparing for the licensing examination, MPJE® candidates should review their individual state regulations.

Medicare Prescription Drug Improvement and Modernization Act of 2003

This complicated act, sometimes referred to as "MMA", was signed into law in December 2003 and is frequently revised.

This Act currently encompasses four programs:

Medicare Part A - Provides hospitalization insurance.

Medicare Part B - Provides medical insurance for physician services.

Medicare Part C - Medicare managed care (Medicare Advantage)

Medicare Part D - Medicare prescription drug program

Some of the terminology used for the MMA programs includes the following:

CMS – Centers for Medicare and Medicaid Services – developed and currently supervises the MMA

MA - Medicare Advantage - plans that cover everything the original Medicare covered but may offer lower costs and extra services.

MA-PD - Medicare Advantage Prescription Drug Plan.

MTM - Medication therapy management.

PDP - Prescription Drug Plan - Medicare prescription drug plans that cover only outpatient drugs and are intended for people in original Medicare who have no other drug coverage. Patients cannot enroll in both a PDP and a MA plan.

TrOOP - True Out-of-Pocket expense to the individual. The sum of an individual's deductible and cost sharing expenses in Medicare Part D.

Another form of managed care is the HMOs, which require that you generally utilize only doctors and hospitals in the plan's network, except in emergencies or special situations.

Medicare Part D

Since January 2006 Medicare beneficiaries have been able to enroll in the Medicare Part D prescription drug plan (PDP). As part of this program, Medicare contracts with private insurance companies to provide drug-only coverage OR coverage through Medicare Advantage local and regional managed care plans, the MA-PD. The cost to the beneficiary depends on the beneficiary's income. If the beneficiary is not in a low-income category, they will pay a monthly premium, have an annual deductible, and have co-payment responsibilities. The PDP benefits include the cost of any prescription drug, biological product, and insulin if it is presently covered by Medicaid and is intended for a medically accepted indication.

Note

Examination questions concerning dollar amounts are NOT likely to be asked on the MPJE® since the amounts may vary among plan providers and they will likely change every year.

The premiums, deductibles, and percentages are based upon an individual. Therefore, a husband and wife must each have their own plans. Part D deductibles may be reduced or waived by a health insurance company, but a company may charge a higher premium for this benefit. Other insurance company options include charging a higher co-payment. Co-payments (co-pays) may be based on a three or four level tier system developed by each health coinsurance company. The tiers often consist of:

Tier 1: least expensive generic drug

Tier 2: preferred brand name drug

Tier 3: non-preferred brand name drug

Tier 4: rarer, high cost drugs

Once the beneficiary has enrolled, the premium and deductible cannot change between January 1 and December 31. The co-pay amount may change if the drug is moved to another tier. The beneficiary may change plans only once a year unless he/she moves out of the plan's area, into a nursing home, or the plan stops service in the area.

The Medicare Part D coverage gap, often coined the "Medicare donut hole", describes the financial gap between the Part D Rx initial coverage limit and the catastrophic-coverage threshold. This gap is when the patient pays the largest amount for prescriptions until reaching the the catastrophic-coverage level. For example, in 2015, the patient paid a $320 deductible then Part D covered until drug expenses reached $2960 which included payments by both the patient (TrOOP) and the insurance company. During the gap limit (the donut hole) the patient had to pay most of the cost (but with 50% discount on brand-name drugs and 35% discount for generics). When out-of-pocket reaches $4,700, the plan paid for most costs.

Patients may choose plans that either reduce or eliminate the donut hole. By 2020 the donut hole is planned to be completely phased out.

Other provisions of Medicare programs include the following:

1. All Rx benefits programs must accept participation from any pharmacy that agrees to the terms and conditions of their drug plan. This is referred to as the "any willing provider clause".
2. The sponsors cannot require beneficiaries to obtain their prescriptions through mail-order pharmacies.
3. Larger quantities, including 90-day supplies of long-term drugs, may be obtained at the participating local pharmacy.
4. If a brand-name product is dispensed, the patient must be informed of the availability of lower-cost generic versions of the drug.
5. Pharmacists are eligible to receive payment from Medicare for providing medication therapy management (MTM), if the patient is enrolled in Medicare Part D.
6. Each drug plan sponsor must establish medication therapy management (MTM) programs for enrolled individuals having high drug costs resulting from multiple chronic conditions such as asthma, diabetes, hypertension, hyperlipidemia, etc.
7. Importation of drugs from Canada and some other countries may be permitted if the HHS certifies that the importation poses no additional risk to the public health.
8. Explicitly blocking the use of Medicare's purchasing power

to negotiate prices with pharmaceutical manufacturers to obtain lower cost drugs for the elderly and disabled.

9. Bringing higher reimbursement prices paid by Medicare into a lower range. The manufacturer-reported AWP will be phased out in favor of an "ASP" – average sales price. This value will be between the actual acquisition price (AAP) paid and the present AWP.

10. Preventing a drug company from filing multiple 30-month stays to prevent competing companies from marketing a generic version of a drug product.

11. Allowing multiple manufacturers of a generic product to obtain a 180 day exclusivity period if they file their applications on the first day of eligibility.

Items 10 and 11 are intended to close loopholes in the Drug Price Competition and Patent-Term Restoration Act of 1984 (Hatch-Waxman Amendment) discussed in Section B.

In 2008 Medicare Part D began to cover the cost of vaccines and their administration, which formerly was covered by Part B.

All sponsors must establish a method to identify beneficiaries with "multiple chronic diseases" and/or those receiving multiple drugs under the Part D plan. Plans must utilize the assistance of physicians and pharmacists to create services that will help beneficiaries who are likely to incur high yearly costs.

Formulary Requirements

All standard plans must include drugs within all the therapeutic categories and classes developed by the USP. Companies desiring to develop their own formularies must have a Pharmacy and Therapeutics (P & T) Committee with the majority of members comprised of practicing physicians and pharmacists. Insurers do NOT have to include **all** drugs within each category. However, there are six drug classes that do require that most drug products be included.

These categories are:

- anticonvulsants
- antidepressants
- antineoplastics
- antipsychotics
- antiretrovirals
- immunosuppressants

Drugs in any category must be for a medically accepted indication. Therefore, research drugs are not covered but "off-label" use drugs may be acceptable. The insurer may change or remove specific drugs after giving timely notice to enrollees and health professionals. Plans may alter their therapeutic categories and classes of drugs only at the beginning of each plan year unless a change is needed to accommodate newly approved drugs or new uses of an existing drug. Maintenance changes to formularies such as removing a branded drug and replacing it with a newly available generic is allowed at any time. Advance notice must be given to the CMS for its approval. Pharmacies and beneficiaries must also be notified before changes are made. If a specific drug is not covered by a plan, the patients may appeal for exceptions if his/her doctor can show that the non-formulary drug is medically necessary.

Also, under the standard Part D plans, the following groups of drugs are generally not covered:

- barbiturates
- benzodiazepines
- weight loss or weight gain drugs
- hair growth drugs
- drugs that increase fertility
- prescription vitamins except prenatal and fluoride products
- outpatient drugs for which the manufacturer requires monitoring

Enhanced Part D plans may cover some of the above drugs; most likely with an increased premium.

Formulary changes by plans, such as drug removal or reduction to a less favorable tier must be done with CMS approval. A 60-day notice must be given to CMS, state prescription plans, pharmacies, and plan enrollees. The exception is a formulary drug that has a new black-box warning, which may be removed at any time. If an enrollee is taking the drug being "switched", he or she must be allowed to obtain the drug without penalty for the rest of the plan year.

Prescriptions Access at "out-of-network" Pharmacies

Sponsors of Part D plans must ensure that the beneficiary will be able to obtain prescription drugs when traveling outside of the geographic area of their pharmacy or when the pharmacy they normally use is either closed or the drug is out of stock.

When it is necessary to patronize an "out-of-network pharmacy", the beneficiary must pay the new pharmacy's usual and customary price when purchasing the prescription. The beneficiary will then submit a claim to their plan for reimbursement. The beneficiary is responsible for any difference in the new pharmacy's charge and that allowed by the plan sponsor.

Medicare Enrollment

Those individuals who become eligible for Medicare have an initial enrollment period that begins three months before and lasts three months after the month of their birthday. In other words, a time span of seven months. After enrollment, clients are "locked" into their specific plan until the next general enrollment period. At that time, they may switch to another plan. Failure to enroll in a plan may result in a late-enrollment penalty.

A beneficiary's monthly premium is based upon the individual coverage they have chosen and may be paid directly each month or deducted from monthly Social Security checks.

Anyone enrolling in Medicare may no longer contribute to health savings accounts (HSAs). This is a medical savings account intended to ease the cost of medical care for working individuals. It is available to taxpayers in the United States who are enrolled in a high-deductible health plan (HDHP). The funds contributed to such an account are not subject to federal income tax at the time of deposit.

Medigap

A Medigap policy is health insurance sold by private insurance companies to fill the "gaps" in the original Medicare Plan coverage. It is sometimes referred to as Medicare Supplemental Insurance. Health insurance companies are not permitted to sell new Medigap policies that cover drugs. However, people who already have such policies may keep them. Medigap plans without drug coverage may still be sold. Medigap supplementary insurance covers some out-of-pocket expenses not paid by original Medicare.

There are about 12 different types of Medigap policies available. These policies must follow federal and state laws. A Medigap policy must be clearly identified on the cover as "Medicare Supplement Insurance." Each policy has a different set of basic and extra benefits.

The Medication Therapy Management (MTM) Program

Medication therapy management, also referred to as MTM, is a term used to describe a broad range of health care services provided by pharmacists. It is defined as a service or group of services that optimize therapeutic outcomes for individual patients. Medication therapy management services include medication therapy reviews, pharmacotherapy consults, anticoagulation management, immunizations, health and wellness programs and many other clinical services.

Pharmacists generally provide medication therapy management to help patients get the greatest benefits from their medications by actively managing drug therapy and by identifying, preventing and resolving medication-related problems.

The Centers for Medicare and Medicaid Services (CMS) has stated that MTM programs must "evolve and become a cornerstone of the Medicare prescription drug benefit". CMS has committed itself to increasing access to MTM and reducing eligibility restrictions for beneficiaries. As of 2016, CMS has increased requirements for Part D sponsors to provide MTM programs. Included in these requirements are the following:

- Part D sponsors must automatically enroll qualified beneficiaries, unless they opt-out.
- Beneficiaries must be targeted for enrollment at least quarterly. Part D sponsors must target beneficiaries who
  - — have multiple chronic disease states – usually 2-3 or more.
  - — are taking many Part D medications – sponsors may set the minimum number of drugs from 2 to 8.
  - — are predicted to incur a predetermined annual cost from Part D medications. NOTE: the cost threshold for 2016 is $3507 per year.
- Sponsors cannot require more than three chronic illness and MUST target at least four of the following seven core chronic disease states:
  - — Hypertension
  - — Heart failure
  - — Diabetes
  - — Dyslipidemia
  - — Respiratory disease (e.g. asthma, COPD, etc.)

- Bone disease – arthritis (e.g. osteoporosis, osteoarthritis, rheumatoid arthritis, etc.)
- Mental health (e.g. schizophrenia, depression, bipolar disorder, etc.)

- Offer interventions for beneficiaries and prescribers
- Report specific outcomes data to CMS. Reports should include
  - The number of CMRs
  - The number of targeted medication reviews
  - The number of prescriber interventions
  - The change(s) in therapy directly resulting from the MTM interventions.
- Minimum interventions must include
  - Comprehensive medication review (CMR) – this must include a review of medications, offering interactive consultation, and providing consultation summaries face-to-face or by telephone.

> **Note**
>
> Sponsors are not required to provide interactive consultations to long term care (LTC) residents.

  - Targeted medication review – may be done person-to-person or by computer.
  - Reviews must be done at least quarterly for each participating beneficiary.
  - Interventions targeted to prescribers may be either passive (fax, mail, etc.) or interactive.
- Sponsors may include passive interventions such as
  - Educational newsletters

— Drug utilization review (DUR) edits

— Refill reminders

— Medication lists

> ***Note***
>
> The MMA will undoubtedly be subject to changes and various interpretations by the Administration, Congress, and other bodies over the next few years. Consult the most recent sources for changes.

Sample Questions

1. Which of the following population(s) is (are) covered under the MMA?

   I. Medicare beneficiaries

   II. Medicaid beneficiaries

   III. nongovernmental employees

   (A) I only (B) III only (C) I and II only
   (D) II and III only (E) I, II, and III

2. At what intervals may a patient with a Medicare PDP or MA-PD card change his/her provider?

   (A) Every month

   (B) Every 6 months

   (C) Once a year

   (D) Whenever he/she desires

   (E) Never

3. A pharmacy providing services under MMA may establish a formulary limiting the drugs to which of the following?

   (A) The top 200 frequently dispensed drugs
   (B) Only drugs available generically
   (C) Only brand-name drugs
   (D) 100 brand-name drugs plus their equivalent generic products
   (E) At least one drug from each of 8 therapeutic categories

4. Which of the following is (are) NOT permissible under the MMA?

   I. Requiring a beneficiary to use a mail order pharmacy.
   II. Requiring a beneficiary to use a mail order pharmacy for 90-day supplies of a maintenance drug.
   III. Changing the price of a drug product one month after establishing a certain price

   (A) I only (B) III only (C) I and II only
   (D) II and III only (E) I, II, and III

5. Which one of the following acronyms will eventually replace the AWP when calculating drug product prices under the MMA?

   (A) ASP (B) BDP (C) ESP (D) NARD (E) SP

6. The term "donut hole" refers to which of the following situations?

   (A) Prescription drug costs to the beneficiary before reaching the catastrophic coverage
   (B) The period of time during which a person may enroll in Plan D
   (C) The period of time during which a beneficiary may change health insurance companies

(D) The portion of prescription drug costs charged to the insurance company

(E) A dollar range in which the beneficiary must pay for all prescription drugs

7. Which one of the following is TRUE for a client who becomes eligible for Medicare Plan D on April 1st of the present year?

   (A) Cannot enroll into the program until her next birthday

   (B) May enroll at anytime without a penalty

   (C) Must enroll within a certain time span without a penalty

   (D) Must wait until January 1st of the following year

   (E) May sign up immediately but benefits will not start until April of the following year

8. An individual will become eligible for Medicare Plan D on July 4th of a certain year. Which of the following is the maximum time span for her to enroll in a PDP without penalty?

   (A) July 4th to Dec 31st

   (B) April 1st to Oct 31st

   (C) Jan 1st to December 31st

   (D) July 1st to July 31st

   (E) July 1st to September 31st

9. When reviewing the choices of drugs covered in various Plan D programs, a beneficiary is likely to find only a limited choice of brand name products in which of the following categories of drugs?

   (A) anticonvulsants

   (B) antidepressants

   (C) antihyperlipidemics

   (D) antineoplastics

   (E) antipsychotics

10. Mrs Stenson is about to file for social security as she is turning 65. Into which of the following portions of Medicare will she automatically be enrolled?

(A) A only (B) B only (C) A and B
(D) A and D (E) B and D

11. Which group of the following individuals are ineligible to contribute to health savings accounts (HSAs)?

(A) enrolled in Medicare

(B) gross earnings over $100,000

(C) gross earnings over $200,000

(D) gross earnings over $500,000

(E) gross earnings over $1 million

12. When a patient asks who has to pay the expense designated as TrOOP, the pharmacist should state it is the:

(A) Drug company

(B) Federal government

(C) Insurance company

(D) Patient

(E) State government

Answers:

(1) A (2) C (3) E (4) C (5) A (6) E (7) C (8) B (9) C (10) C (11) A (12) D

Section E

Bringing New Drugs to Market

Investigational New Drug Application (IND)

Before a new drug is marketed, a sponsor (usually a manufacturer) has to complete an extensive testing process to assure that the new drug will be safe and effective for what it is claimed to do. The Investigational New Drug Application (IND) is the first application form that a sponsor must submit to the FDA before a drug may be administered to humans. The requirement for an IND approval is intended to protect both the rights and safety of humans in whom the drug will be tested.

While most IND sponsors are pharmaceutical companies, it is possible for a medical researcher, academic personnel, or organizations, either public or private, to submit INDs. Once an IND has been submitted, the FDA has 30 days in which to decide whether the investigational drug is suitable for testing.

Virtually all of the information collected by the sponsor, especially from preclinical (animal) studies, which reflect on both the use and safety of the proposed investigational drug, is submitted to the FDA as part of the IND application. In addition, the sponsor must provide complete descriptions of the methodology (clinical protocols) to be used in testing the drugs in humans.

Clinical Trials

After the FDA approves an IND, the sponsor may initiate clinical (human) trials. There are three phases before the final approval of the drug may be provided, and one additional phase after the drug product has been marketed. The drug must satisfactorily complete each phase before it can progress to the next.

— Phase 1 - A small group of healthy individuals is given the drug. The primary purpose of this phase is to evaluate the drug's toxicological, pharmacokinetic and pharmacological properties, as well as to assess the safety of the drug in humans.

— Phase 2 - A larger group (100 or more) of patients that have the disease or symptoms of the condition to be treated by the drug is given the new drug. The purpose of this phase is to determine the effectiveness of the drug and to obtain information about adequate dosage, relative safety, and adverse effects.

— Phase 3 - Large groups of patients (sometimes thousands) in several geographical locations are part of controlled clinical studies. The purpose of this phase is to obtain data concerning the drug's effectiveness as compared to a control group that receives a placebo. Most Phase 3 studies are double-blinded (i.e. neither the patient or investigator knows whether the drug or placebo is being given until after the study has been completed).

Phase 1 and 2 studies are usually conducted under the direct supervision of the sponsoring company while Phase 3 studies usually involve testing performed at remote and varied clinical sites by independent investigators. Obviously Phase 3 studies are the most costly and take an extended period of time to complete. In each of these first three phases the patient or their representative must provide informed consent, i.e. they must agree to be subjects in the testing program after having been advised of the potential risks.

Treatment Investigational New Drugs

Treatment INDs allow the administration of an investigational new drug to patients that have not been enrolled in the new drug's clinical trials program. These patients must be in an imminent life-threatening stage of an illness for which there is presently no cure or where the presently used drugs do not appear to be effective. Examples of such diseases might be advanced stages of AIDS, some cancers, Alzheimer's disease, and Parkinson's disease.

The company developing the drug must have presented data outlining the drug's safety and efficacy, and the drug must be in either Phase 2 or 3 of clinical trials. If the drug is being considered as a Treatment IND candidate, a "treatment protocol" must be submitted to the FDA, which describes its proposed use in the designated patients.

The New Drug Application (NDA) Process

Once sufficient data concerning drug efficacy, toxicity, stability, production methods, packaging and the data from numerous clinical trials on patients have been collected, a new drug application may be submitted to the FDA for review. If the FDA reviewers are satisfied with the accuracy and completeness of the data from the clinical trials (Phases 1, 2 and 3), the NDA is approved and the NDA will be "on file" at the FDA. At this point, the manufacturer may market the new drug product.

The NDA often consists of thousands of pages of data and information and is very costly and time-consuming to prepare. Once submitted, the FDA generally reviews the application for at least six months and provides experts and other interested parties the opportunity to comment on the submission.

After the drug product is marketed, Phase 4 studies are conducted. This is the post-marketing surveillance of the drug. During this period, health professionals are encouraged to report any problems with the drug, especially adverse effects experienced when the drug is used. The drug manufacturer must also submit yearly reports concerning new information and field reports concerning the drug product. The FDA utilizes Phase 4 data to determine whether or not a product should remain on the market.

FDA Expedited Review Programs

The U.S. Food and Drug Administration (FDA) attempts to review all drugs efficiently, but gives special consideration to therapies that treat serious or life-threatening diseases or have the potential to provide unusually large benefits to patients. The following are the four ways used by FDA to speed the development and availability of drugs that are intended to treat serious or life-threatening conditions.

Priority Review

- Used for Biologics License Application (BLA) or New Drug Application (NDA) submission
- Reduces a drug's FDA review period from ten months to six
- Drugs qualifying for Fast Track, Breakthrough Therapy, and Accelerated Approval can also be eligible for Priority Review

Fast Track

- May be requested for Investigational New Drug (IND) application and prior to BLA or NDA submission
- Intended for drugs that address unmet medical need by either treating a condition for which no other treatment exists or drugs that offer substantial benefit over existing treatment
- Sponsors get extra opportunities to meet with FDA to discuss study design and how to best expedite the drug development
- Sponsors may have early reviews of their product marketing before the complete application has been submitted

Breakthrough Therapy

- May be requested as early as IND application and preferably prior to end-of-Phase II meeting
- Similar to Fast Track, but Breakthrough drugs must show early clinical evidence of substantial improvement over existing therapies
- Same benefits as Fast Track, with an even greater emphasis on early meetings and coordination with experienced and senior FDA personnel
- Breakthrough drugs can sometimes skip portions of the standard FDA review process without compromising safety and efficacy standards

Accelerated Approval

- Sponsors should discuss Accelerated Approval with FDA during development
- Intended for drugs with long-term endpoints, such as increased survival or decreased morbidity, that are difficult to measure efficiently in trials
- Allows approval based on easily measured outcomes that are reasonably likely to predict clinical benefit (e.g. tumor shrinkage for survival benefit in some instances of cancer)
- Sponsors are required to confirm a drug's efficacy in post-market clinical trials
- Priority Review, Fast Track, and Breakthrough drugs can also be eligible for Accelerated Approval

Abbreviated New Drug Application (ANDA)

Before any new drug may be placed on the market, the innovator company must submit the data described for INDs and NDAs.

Usually the innovator pharmaceutical company will have patent protection for their drug entity. However, once the patent expires, other companies may wish to introduce the drug under the drug's generic name only or as a brand name product. Rather than requiring the secondary companies to submit a complete NDA, the FDA will permit an Abbreviated New Drug Application (ANDA) to be submitted. These submissions require less data, but do require proof that the new drug product's pharmacokinetic properties, its bioavailability, and clinical activity are similar to that of the innovator's drug product.

The first applicant to complete a formal review showing that its generic product is biologically equivalent to the brand name product will be rewarded with six months of exclusive rights to sell the generic.

An important issue related to generic drugs is whether generic drug companies can be sued if a drug product they market is claimed to be defectively designed or for failing to warn about a drug's dangers because the generic company must use the same safety label as the brand-name version.

In 2011 and again in 2013 the U.S. Supreme Court ruled that generic companies could not be sued for such issues. These issues will undoubtedly continue to be debated in the years to come because generic drugs constitute about 80% of all prescriptions filled in the U.S.

Supplemental New Drug Application (SNDA)

After marketing a drug product, the manufacturer may desire to make some changes in the drug's synthesis, production procedures or manufacturing locations, packaging, labeling, etc. Rather than submit an NDA, the company may submit a Supplemental New Drug Application (SNDA). This abbreviated application permits desired changes to be implemented.

Note

To distinguish between the necessity for an ANDA versus a SNDA, just picture that any changes or additions made by the company that filed the original NDA will probably require a Supplemental New Drug Application. Examples would include adding a new dosage form, tablet strength, or therapeutic use for the original drug. However, if another company is submitting data for a drug product similar to the drug in the original NDA, it will most likely need to file an Abbreviated New Drug Application.

FDA Classification System for New Drugs

During the drug approval process, the FDA classifies new drugs based on their chemical and therapeutic characteristics. Health professionals employ these ratings to assess the potential value of a new drug.

Therapeutic Classification

- **Type P** - Indicates that the drug represents a major therapeutic gain because there are no other effective drugs available for treating a particular illness or because it has significant advantages compared to currently marketed drugs. Drugs classified as Type P are often given a priority review. (Hint: Think "P" = priority)
- **Type S** - Indicates that the drug is similar to other drugs on the market. Such drugs will generally undergo a standard review. (Hint: Think "S" = standard or similar)

Note

A Type P drug will usually be reviewed more rapidly than a Type S drug and will, therefore, generally be marketed sooner, if approved by the FDA.

Chemical Classification

- **Type 1** - Indicates a new molecular structure, different from existing drugs, that may be used for the same therapeutic purpose. The drug must not be presently marketed in the United States.
- **Type 2** - Indicates that the drug is a new derivative of a molecular structure already approved in the United States; for example a new salt or ester of an existing drug.
- **Type 3** - Indicates that the drug is a new formulation of a drug already marketed in the US.
- **Type 4** - Indicates that the product is a new combination of two or more drugs.
- **Type 5** - Indicates that a drug is being manufactured by a new company.
- **Type 6** - Indicates a new therapeutic indication for a drug already approved.

Note

It is probably NOT necessary to memorize the six chemical classification types. Instead, just remember that Type 1 is the best type since a new, unique drug is being placed on the market. Also remember that Type 6 is important since it will generally increase the sales and use of a drug product already on the market.

To further complicate matters, some drugs are also classified as:

- **Type AA** - Indicates a drug with potential use for AIDS or HIV- related disease; such drugs are often given fast-track status for potential approval.
- **Type E** - Indicates a drug for a life-threatening or severely debilitating disease; these drugs are also given a priority review and may be used in patients in imminent danger of death.
- **Type F** - Indicates a drug that has been placed on hold until submitted data has been further validated.
- **Type N** - Indicates a drug that is being considered for nonprescription status.
- **Type V** - Indicates a drug that is being considered for "orphan drug" status.

Orphan Drugs

An orphan drug is one that would be difficult for a company to develop into a profitable product because the cost of the NDA process would exceed the anticipated market sales. Usually these drugs are marketed for the treatment of diseases that affect a relatively small patient population.

Rare diseases or conditions are considered to be those that affect fewer than 200,000 persons in the US. In some cases, orphan drug status may be given to a product that will be useful for more persons if there is no reasonable expectation that cost of development of the product will be recovered by sales of the drug.

The Orphan Drug Act of 1983 encourages companies to develop orphan drugs by giving them incentives such as tax relief, exclusive marketing rights, and faster NDA approval.

Vaccines for Children Program (VCP)

The Vaccines For Children (VFC) program is a federally funded program. It provides for administration of 16 vaccines at no cost to children who might not otherwise be vaccinated because of inability to pay. CDC buys vaccines at a discount and distributes them to state health departments and certain local and territorial public health agencies. These agencies then distribute them at no charge to those private physicians' offices and public health clinics registered as VFC providers.

Sample Questions

1. How many phases of clinical testing must be conducted before a new drug application may be submitted to the FDA?

   (A) 2 (B) 3 (C) 4 (D) 5 (E) 8

2. The prime purpose of Phase 1 clinical trials is to evaluate the drug's

   (A) therapeutic index
   (B) safety
   (C) adverse effects in diseased patients
   (D) efficacy in diseased patients
   (E) marketability

3. Phase 1 clinical trials involve subjects that

   (A) are healthy humans without the disease
   (B) are lower species of animals
   (C) are primates
   (D) are in a state of disease remission
   (E) have active cases of a disease

4. A clinical pharmacist in a hospital setting is most likely to participate in which phase of pre-marketing clinical testing?

   (A) 1 (B) 3 (C) 5 (D) 6 (E) 8

5. A pharmaceutical company plans to market a generic version of a drug product whose patent has expired. Which type of documentation must be submitted to the FDA?

(A) IND (B) NDA (C) ANDA
(D) SNDA (E) Letter of intent

6. A pharmaceutical company that wishes to lengthen the expiration date of a drug product based upon additional stability data should submit to the FDA a(n):

(A) IND (B) NDA (C) ANDA
(D) SNDA (E) Letter of Intent

7. Post-marketing surveillance of a new drug product is sometimes referred to as the Phase _____ clinical trial.

(A) 1 (B) 2 (C) 3 (D) 4 (E) 5

8. Which one of the following designations indicates that a new drug possesses significant advancement over present drug therapy?

(A) Type 1 (B) Type 2 (C) Type 4
(D) Type A (E) Type AB

9. An orphan drug is one that has:

(A) been removed from the market because of toxicity.
(B) been discontinued because of poor sales.
(C) special economical incentives for the manufacturer.
(D) a low therapeutic index.
(E) been developed and imported from a foreign country.

10. Some new drug applications are granted a "Type P" status by the FDA. This status implies that the drug

(A) is for parenteral use.
(B) will be packaged in a novel container.
(C) will receive a low priority (passive) review.
(D) is intended for patients with AIDS.
(E) will receive a priority review of the NDA.

11. For which one of the following purposes may a NDA be granted a "Type P" status?
    (A) pediatric use
    (B) a novel packaging container
    (C) intended for a patient with AIDS
    (D) parenteral administration
    (E) a priority review

12. Which one of the following is NOT recognized by the FDA as a drug approval review designation?
    (A) accelerated approval
    (B) breakthrough drug approval
    (C) fast track
    (D) double fast tract
    (E) priority review

13. Which is the designation of the first clinical trial phase that assesses a drug's efficacy?
    (A) 1 (B) 2 (C) 3 (D) 4 (E) 5

Answers:

(1) B (2) B (3) A (4) B (5) C (6) D (7) D
(8) A (9) C (10) E (11) E (12) D (13) B

Section F

Requirements for Marketed Drug Products

Naming New Drugs

During the research phases of drug development, the pharmaceutical manufacturer will probably identify an investigational drug by a code name, such as WIN 2306. This avoids the use of the burdensome, long chemical name. Once the drug nears its final approval, a specific name known as the non-proprietary or generic name must be established. The company may also select a trade name or brand name for the drug to encourage prescriber recognition of that company's specific product.

The responsibility for designating a nonproprietary or generic name for a new drug belongs to the United States Adopted Names Council (USAN). This group is sponsored by the American Medical Association (AMA), American Pharmacists Association (APhA), and the United States Pharmacopeial Convention (USPC). However, the Secretary of Human Health Services (HHS) must grant final approval for any drug name. The Secretary may also require the change of a drug name if there appears to be confusion because of two similar drug names (either generic or brand name products).

A distinctive generic name, proprietary name, or USAN is assigned to each new drug based on the following criteria:

- The name should be short, distinctive, and not likely to be confused with other existing names.
- The name should provide some indication of the therapeutic or chemical class to which the drug belongs.

Patent Protection

There are considerable costs and time delays when a company develops a new drug and submits a New Drug Application (NDA). In order to allow the company to recover these costs, Congress passed an act to guarantee the innovator company a minimum time period for patent protection before generic versions of the drug product could be marketed.

Up to 1984, innovator companies had a 17-year period of exclusive patent rights, including the time that elapsed during the development period and the FDA review process. The Drug Price Competition and Patent-Term Restoration Act of 1984, also known as the Waxman-Hatch Amendment, represents a compromise affecting major drug manufacturers and generic companies. The major drug manufacturers were granted longer patent protection (up to an extra five years) while the manufacturers of generic drugs were provided with easier access to approval of their drug applications. The generic manufacturer is relieved of proving the safety and efficacy of their drug through clinical studies. Instead, the drug must be shown to be bioequivalent to the innovator's drug product. In June 2005 the Supreme Court ruled that drug makers do not have to wait until a patent expires before conducting basic research. Thus, a company could conduct studies on a drug protected by another company's patent.

In order to encourage clinical studies of drugs in the pediatric population, the Secretary of HHS may request that such studies be performed if the drug has yet to be approved and may be of value in pediatric patients. An incentive to the pharmaceutical company is an extension of patent protection, usually an additional 6 months. These studies may also be conducted for already marketed drugs and drug products intended for the treatment of rare diseases or symptoms.

National Drug Code (NDC)

The NDC is a numbering system that aids in identifying a drug product. Third party payers also employ NDC numbers to identify products for reimbursement.

The NDC of a specific drug product contains ten or eleven digits. For example, a number may be:

1 0 7 4	0 1 2 8	0 4
(manufacturer)	(ID of specific drug)	(ID of package)

Each manufacturer has its own number which has been assigned to them by the FDA. This number is known as the "labeler's code". Each company can then establish its own identification numbers, known as "product codes", for a specific drug, its strength, and dosage form. That is, one company might designate warfarin 10 mg tablets as 0128 and another company's warfarin 10 mg tablets may be assigned the number 0045. The last two digits usually indicate the package characteristic such as 04 for blister packs or 02 for bottles of 100 tablets.

Newer drug products have either 10 or 11 digit NDC numbers, of which the first five represent the manufacturer and the remaining digits represent the drug and package.

The NDC Directory is a publication that contains listings of NDC numbers and their identity. Other books, such as the *Red Book* and the *Blue Book*, as well as the *National Drug Code Directory*, available at the FDA website, have NDC numbers and their equivalents listed.

All prescription drugs marketed in the United States must have NDC numbers. While placing the NDC number on the package labeling is not mandatory, most companies do so. The NDC number also does not have to appear on individual dosage units nor is there any federal law requiring that NDC numbers appear on prescription labels. However, the NDC serves as a convenient identification tool when transferring information electronically; for example, when requesting reimbursement or ordering drug products.

If a manufacturer discontinues a product, the NDC number may be reassigned to another drug product provided that at least five years has elapsed from the last commercial shipment of the discontinued drug product.

Good Manufacturing Practice (GMP)

Current Good Manufacturing Practice (GMP) is a set of regulations that specify the minimum standards required to manufacture pharmaceutical products in the US. They are designed to assure safety and quality of pharmaceuticals. Compliance with these regulations is a responsibility of pharmaceutical manufacturers.

While there are many requirements under GMP regulations, this material is unlikely to be tested on the MPJE®. Candidates should, however, be aware that manufacturers must be registered with the FDA and they must describe their manufacturing and production processes as part of the NDA process. The FDA inspects the drug manufacturer's facilities approximately once every two years to determine compliance with GMPs, unless a prior history of deficiencies indicates the need for more frequent visits.

Bad Advertising

In 2010, the FDA's Division of Drug Marketing, Advertising, and Communications (DDMAC), now renamed as Office of Prescription Drug Promotion ("OPDP"), started its Bad Ad Program. Bad advertising about prescription drugs may be reported to the OPDP by e-mailing a summary of an incident to BadAd@ fda.gov or by calling 301-796-1200. Its purpose is to educate health care providers about misleading or inaccurate promotion of prescription drugs by companies. It also solicits help from health care providers in identifying and reporting such activities. Bad advertising about prescription drugs may be reported to the OPDP by e-mailing a summary of an incident to BadAd@fda.gov or by calling 301-796-1200.

Question

One purpose of the FDA's section known as OPDP is to receive reports concerning:

(A) bad or misleading advertisements

(B) drug interactions

(C) mislabeled drug products

(D) overpriced prescription drugs

(E) unusual allergies

Answer = (A)

Adulteration versus Misbranding of Products

The distinction between the terms "adulteration" and "misbranding" is important to regulatory bodies when attempting to remove a product from the market. Adulteration refers to the composition of a product while misbranding refers to the labeling. A product is considered to be adulterated if:

- it contains in whole or in part any filthy, putrid, or decomposed substance.
- it has been prepared, packaged, or held under unsanitary conditions where it may have been contaminated.
- it has been manufactured under conditions that do not meet the standards of Good Manufacturing Practice (GMPs).
- it contains an unapproved color additive.
- it contains a drug recognized in official compendia, but its strength, purity or quality is lower than the official standards.
- its container is composed of a deleterious substance that may enter (leach) into the product contents.

- it contains a drug not recognized in official compendia, but its strength, quality, or purity is lower than that listed on the label.
- it contains any ingredient as a substitute for the active drug.

Drugs or drug products that are sold, dispensed, or distributed in violation of the labeling requirements are considered misbranded. A drug or drug product is considered to be misbranded if the labeling

- is false or misleading.
- is missing either the name or location of the manufacturer, packer, or distributor.
- does not contain a word, statement or other information required by law to be displayed in a prominent, readable manner.
- does not include the established name of the active drug .
- does not have each active drug ingredient identified.
- does not state "Rx only" if the drug is available only by prescription. (However, when dispensing to a consumer, the prescription label does not have to state "Rx only").
- does not contain a precautionary statement for a drug product that is subject to deterioration.
- is missing the quantity of the container contents (e.g. a numerical count of 100, net weight of 50 g, or a net volume of 4 fluid ounces).
- has inadequate directions for use of nonprescription drugs or does not include appropriate warnings required to protect those using the medication or packaging.
- is not in accordance with USP/NF specifications.
- offers the sale of a drug under the name of another drug.

> ***Note***
>
> It is considered misbranding if a pharmacy dispenses a prescription-only drug without a legal prescription or an authorized refill.

Product Labeling

The term "label" refers to written, printed, or graphic matter appearing on the immediate container of a drug product. If there is an outside package, any word, statement, or other information present on the immediate container must also appear on the outside package.

The term "labeling" refers to either:

- the information printed on the label and outside package of a drug product. It refers to all labels and other written, printed, or graphic matter either on the product, its container, its wrapper, or accompanying the product. Thus, the prescription drug product insert is considered part of the labeling.
- the information printed by the pharmacist on the prescription label for a drug product being dispensed. (NOTE: The prescription label will be discussed later).

While the original Food, Drug, and Cosmetic Act of 1938 specified that all drug products had to be labeled with "adequate directions for use", the Durham-Humphrey Amendment of 1951 clarified these requirements. It states that drugs do NOT have to have adequate directions for use IF they are intended for dispensing by pharmacists, provided that they contain the legend "Caution: Federal law prohibits dispensing without a prescription". In 1997 this required statement was simplified to read "Rx only".

Labeling Requirements for Manufacturer's Containers

Federal law requires that the following information appear on manufacturer's containers of drug products:

- Name and address of the manufacturer, packer, or distributor.
- Established name of the drug or drug product.
- The net quantity (weight, quantity, or dosage units) in the package.
- The weight of each active ingredient contained in each dosage unit (e.g. 10 mg or 2 mg/5 mL). An additional requirement for electrolyte replacement therapy is inclusion of the electrolyte concentration in terms of milliequivalents (mEq).
- The federal legend "Caution: Federal law prohibits dispensing without a prescription" or the more recent version, "Rx only".
- If dosage units are not taken orally, the specific route or routes of administration must be stated (e.g. for IM or subcutaneous injection).
- Special storage directions, if appropriate.
- Manufacturer's control or lot number.
- The expiration date established by the manufacturer.

If these labeling guidelines are not meticulously adhered to, the product may be considered misbranded.

> ***Note***
>
> The term "adequate directions for use" in federal laws dealing with OTC labeling means that sufficient information is provided on the labeling so that a layperson could use the product safely.

Inactive Ingredients on Labels

Stating the names of inactive adjuvants such as antioxidants, buffers, coloring agents, etc. is considered to be good manufacturing practice. All dosage forms must be labeled to state all added ingredients with the exception of flavors and fragrances. Because of the complexity of ingredients in flavoring agents and perfumes, they may be designated by more common names such as "cherry flavor" or "gardenia aroma".

The additives should be listed alphabetically by name but separate from the list of the therapeutically active ingredients. The names should be those used in the official compendia. If not included in these references, the names may be obtained from other sources. The order of preference for these secondary sources is:

- *USP Dictionary of USAN and International Drug Names*
- CTFA *International Cosmetic Ingredient Dictionary and Handbook*
- *Food Chemicals Codex*

While coloring agents may be present in oral and topical dosage forms, they are expressly prohibited in ophthalmic and parenteral formulations. Ingredients found in some parenteral products, but not necessarily listed on the label, are inert gases that are added to improve stability of the product.

Special Label Warning Requirements

The Food, Drug and Cosmetic Act has special labeling warnings that apply to specific drugs and adjuvants. These include the following:

- **FD&C Yellow No. 5 (tartrazine)** – Presence of this agent must be disclosed and the "precautions" part of the labeling must specify that this agent may cause allergic reactions in some susceptible persons.

- **Aspartame** – Product precautions must specify the following type of warning: Phenylketonurics: Contains phenylalanine __mg per __(dosage unit)
- **Sulfites** – Prescription drugs and wines containing sulfites (usually as a preservative) must contain an allergy warning in the labeling.
- **Mineral Oil** – Requires a warning that specifies that it should only be used at bedtime and that it should not be used in infants except if advised by a physician. The labeling should also discourage the use of mineral oil in pregnancy.
- **Wintergreen oil (methyl salicylate)** – Any product that contains more than 5% of this agent should indicate in the labeling that use other than as directed may be dangerous and that it should be kept out of reach of children.
- **Sodium Phosphate** – Limits the amount of Sodium Phosphate Oral Solution (usually used as a saline laxative) to not more than 90 mL per OTC container.
- **Isoproterenol Inhalation Products** – Require a label warning that indicates that user should not exceed the prescribed dose and that the physician must be contacted if breathing difficulty persists.
- **Ipecac Syrup** – Labeling must include:
  - a boxed statement in red type that states "For emergency use to cause vomiting in poisoning. Before using, call physician, the poison prevention center, or hospital emergency room immediately for advice."
  - the statement "Warning: Keep out of reach of children. Do not use in unconscious persons or for poisoning involving corrosives (lye, strong acids), petroleum distillates such as kerosene, gasoline, cleaning fluids, or for strychnine".
  - the dosage of the medication. The usual dose is one tablespoonful (15 mL) in individuals over one year of age.

In addition, Ipecac Syrup may only be sold in 1 oz. (30 mL) containers.

> **Note**
>
> Caution: remember that Ipecac Fluid Extract is 14 times as potent as Ipecac Syrup.

- **Acetophenetidin (Phenacetin)** – Labeling must include a warning about possible kidney damage when the drug is taken in large amounts or for long periods of time.
- **Salicylates (including aspirin)** – Labeling must include warning regarding Reye's Syndrome.
- **Alcohol Warning** – Internal analgesics and antipyretics including acetaminophen, aspirin, ibuprofen, naproxen, ketoprofen, etc. are required to have a label warning that warns consumers to consult with their physicians before taking these drugs if they consume three or more alcoholic beverages per day.

Package Inserts

Besides the above information, the manufacturer is also required to provide a package insert in prescription drug packages. The information in the package insert must be approved by the FDA and is for informational use only, not for promotional use. The following are required to be included in the package insert:

1. Description of the drug (solubility, chemical characteristics, etc.)
2. Clinical pharmacology
3. Indications and usage
4. Contraindications

5. Warnings
6. Precautions
7. Adverse reactions
8. Potential for abuse or patient dependence
9. Symptoms and treatment of overdose
10. Dosage and administration
11. Available dosage forms of the product
12. Date of the most recent revision of the labeling
13. Recommended or usual dosage

In June 2006 the FDA initiated a new prescription drug information format to improve patient safety. The newly designed package insert, which will be phased in over a period of several years, is intended to provide up-to-date information in an easy-to-read format. The following are some of the major features of the new product insert requirements:

- A new section called Highlights provides immediate access to the most important prescribing information about drug benefits and risks.
- A table of contents that facilitates easy access to detailed safety and efficacy information.
- Inclusion of the date of initial product approval.
- A toll-free number and Internet reporting options are provided to encourage reporting of suspected side effects.

The Highlights include a concise summary of information including

- boxed warnings
- indications and usage
- dosage and administration

Drug manufacturers are also required to list all substantive changes made to the Insert within the past year. Also, the Indications and

Usage plus the Dosage and Administration sections are moved to the beginning of the full prescribing information.

A new section entitled Patient Counseling Information is designed to encourage communication between health professionals and patients. FDA approved patient information concerning a prescription drug product will be printed at the end of the drug label or will accompany the label.

Another source of prescription information is provided on the Internet under the designation of DailyMed. This resource will eventually provide high quality information about most marketed drugs. This Web site,

http://dailymed.nlm.nih.gov/dailymed/about.cfm

provides health information providers and the public with a standard, comprehensive, up-to-date resource of medication content and labeling as found in medication package inserts.

Identification of Commercial Solid Dosage Forms

The Code of Federal Regulations (CFR) requires manufacturers to imprint solid oral dosage forms, whether they are prescription or nonprescription products. The imprint code must permit the identification of both the manufacturer and the specific drug product. There are some exemptions to this requirement. For example, it is impractical to imprint nitroglycerin sublingual tablets.

Prescription Drug Marketing Act 1987

The Prescription Drug Marketing Act of 1987 (sometimes referred to as the "Dingle bill") was enacted to correct the problem of drug diversion from normal distribution channels. It includes provisions that:

- require proper storage of drugs and the maintenance of appropriate distribution records.

- prohibit companies from shipping drugs between states without being registered in the state from which they are being shipped.
- prohibits drugs from being reimported into the United States except by the manufacturer of said drugs.
- requires state licensing of drug wholesalers.
- restricts the sale, purchase or trade of prescription drug samples and bars retail pharmacies from receiving any prescription drug samples. Drug samples obtained by a practitioner may not be delivered to a retail pharmacy, even if they are to be dispensed to that practitioner's patients. In other words, a retail pharmacy may NOT possess any prescription drug samples obtained from ANY source. Possession of such samples would be considered to be drug diversion by the FDA.
- allows the use of starter packs that contain small quantities of drug product, which are distributed free of charge to pharmacies. They are not considered to be samples since they are intended to be distributed by the pharmacy to initiate drug therapy for a patient. Another mechanism of distributing a drug is by providing vouchers or coupons. The voucher may be filled from pharmacy stock at the manufacturer's expense or at a reduced cost to the patient.
- permits pharmacies in health care facilities to receive prescription drug samples only if a licensed prescriber has requested them and if precise records are maintained of their disposition. If such samples are received by the pharmacy, they must be stored separately from the normal drug stock.
- prohibits drug products from being resold by hospitals or other health care facilities if they were purchased at special prices. This prevents a hospital pharmacy from purchasing 1000 packages of an antibiotic at a low price then selling a number of them to a community or chain pharmacy in order to make a profit.

- restricts resale of drug products by hospitals or health care facilities.
- permits practitioners licensed to prescribe to receive drug samples provided that a written request is made with their name, address, medical specialty, signature, name of drug, quantity, manufacturer, and date of request. Drug manufacturers and distributors must keep copies of all requests and keep receipts for three years.
- requires sales representatives to be responsible for all samples and take an annual inventory.
- establishes stiff penalties for violation of this law.

Sample Questions

1. A community pharmacy may fill prescriptions received from a licensed practitioner utilizing a manufacturer's

   I. drug samples

   II. voucher or coupon

   III. starter pack

   (A) I only (B) III only (C) I & II only
   (D) II & III only (E) I, II, & III

2. Commercial oral tablets must have which of the following types of information imprinted on each dosage unit?

   (A) name of the manufacturer
   (B) name and strength of the drug
   (C) a code identifying each of the above
   (D) the expiration date
   (E) date of manufacturing

3. Which of the following statements concerning the National Drug Code (NDC) is (are) true?

I. The NDC must be imprinted on all commercial capsules and tablets.

II. Only drugs that have an approved new drug application on file may have an NDC.

III. The NDC may be used for reimbursement purposes.

(A) I only (B) III only (C) I & II only

(D) II & III only (E) I, II, & III

4. A specific drug product has a NDC of 0137-0145-10. The 0137 in this designation represents:

(A) the generic name of the drug

(B) the location of the company

(C) the name of the company

(D) the trade name of the drug

(E) a unit dose package

5. Manufacturers will place an NDC on package labels for which of the following dosage forms?

I. capsules

II. oral suspensions

III. vials of a parenteral solution

(A) I only (B) III only (C) I & II only

(D) II & III only (E) I, II, & III

6. Which of the following commercial products intended for oral intake must have identification codes on individual dosage units?

   I. Nonprescription tablet products
   II. Prescription tablet products
   III. Prescription capsule dosage forms

   (A) I only (B) III only (C) I & II only
   (D) II & III only (E) I, II, & III

7. The maximum volume of Ipecac Syrup that may be sold without a prescription is:

   (A) 15 mL (B) 30 mL (C) 60 mL
   (D) 120 mL (E) > 120 mL

8. Under which of the following circumstances may Ipecac Syrup be sold without a prescription?

   I. For future use during accidental poisoning.
   II. Only if the household does not have small children.
   III. If the purchaser signs a pharmacy log book.

   (A) I only (B) III only (C) I & II only
   (D) II & III only (E) I, II, & III

9. The label of a bottle of Ipecac Syrup sold OTC for accidental poisoning must:

   I. state that the appropriate dose is the contents of the entire bottle followed by a full glass of water.
   II. provide the telephone number of a poison control center.
   III. must have its warnings printed in red ink.

   (A) I only (B) III only (C) I & II only
   (D) II & III only (E) I, II, & III

10. Under which of the following situations would a drug product be considered misbranded?

    I. The manufacturer cannot prove the sterility of a solution labeled "Sterile Folic Acid Injection".

    II. The concentration of a benzocaine ointment is 2% but is labeled as 5% W/W.

    III. An original bottle labeled 50 tablets contains 30 tablets.

    (A) I only (B) III only (C) I & II only
    (D) II & III only (E) I, II, & III

11. Misbranding would include which of the following?

    I. A pharmacy dispenses a prescription-only drug product without an authorized prescription.

    II. A pharmacy dispenses a refill for a prescription without authorization.

    III. A pharmacy dispenses a drug product which shows evidence of decomposition based on a color change.

    (A) I only (B) III only (C) I & II only
    (D) II & III only (E) I, II, & III

12. According to federal regulations, which of the following must be placed on the prescription label?

    I. The name of the dispensing pharmacy.

    II. A toll-free number for reporting side effects of the product.

    III. The name of the supervising or managing pharmacist.

    (A) I only (B) III only (C) I & II only
    (D) II & III only (E) I, II, & III

Answers:

(1) D (2) C (3) B (4) C (5) E (6) E
(7) B (8) A (9) B (10) B (11) C (12) C

Pregnancy Warnings

Package Inserts generally include pregnancy warnings as part of the "Warnings" section of the Insert. Pregnancy warnings are categorized into five FDA pregnancy categories. These include:

- **Category A** - Indicates that there have been adequate, well-controlled studies in pregnant women that demonstrate no risk to the fetus during the first trimester of pregnancy or during the last two trimesters.
- **Category B** - While adequate, well-controlled studies have not been conducted in pregnant women, animal reproduction studies have failed to demonstrate a risk to the fetus.
- **Category C** - The safety of the drug during human pregnancy has not been determined. Animal studies are either positive for fetal risk or have not been conducted. The drug should not be used in human females unless the potential benefit outweighs the potential risk to the fetus.
- **Category D** - There has been positive evidence of risk to the human fetus mainly based upon adverse reaction data from either investigational or marketing experiences. The drug should be administered only if the potential benefits from the use of the drug in pregnant women may be acceptable despite its potential risks.
- **Category X** - Studies in animals, or reports in pregnant women, indicate that the risk of damage caused by the drug clearly outweighs any possible benefit.

Drugs in Category X are contraindicated in pregnant women or, in most instances, for any woman of childbearing age unless appropriate contraceptive methods are being used. Among the drugs with a Category X rating are isotretinoin, Cytotec, Thalomid and most "statin" drugs used to reduce lipid levels.

Risk Evaluation and Mitigation Strategies (REMS™)

The Food and Drug Administration Amendments Act (FDAAA) of 2007 gave the FDA authority to require an Evaluation and Mitigation Strategy (REMS™) from manufacturers to ensure that the benefits of a drug or biological product outweigh its risks. These requirements include five levels of risk mitigation:

1. **Professional Label and Package Insert**
2. **REMS™ - Medication guide** (MedGuide)
3. **REMS™ - Communication Plan** (may include training videos, protocols, informed consent agreements, etc.)
4. **Elements to Assure Safe use (ETASU)** - these elements may include restrictions on accessing a drug based on the following:
    a. The training or experience of a prescriber
    b. The type of setting that dispenses the drug must demonstrate sufficient training.
    c. The site of care may be specified (e.g. the patient must be admitted to a hospital before receiving the medication).
    d. The patient must show evidence or documentation of safe-use conditions (e.g. access to labs, properly trained practitioners).
    e. The patient must agree to be properly monitored. In some cases the patient must be enrolled in registry.
5. **Implementation System** - These are most often used for drugs with severe adverse event profiles. Such a system generally involves the implementation of a limited distribution and/or access program for the drug. Typical limited distribution systems include the following:
    a. **Open Distribution** - Generally for oral drugs
    b. **Managed Distribution** - Usually for drugs that are used in specialized care sites.

c. **Controlled Distribution** - Usually for drugs that are used by specific types of physicians (e.g oncologists) in a specific practice site.

d. **Restricted Access** - Usually for drugs that require patient registry or are being utilized for treating rare diseases.

Table F-1 lists a sampling of drug products that currently have REMS programs. The columns next to each product name depicts the type(s) of requirements assigned to the product.

Since the REMS™ list is modified frequently, the FDA has provided a website called REMS™@FDA, which can be found at http://www.accessdata.fda.gov/scripts/cder/rems/index.cfm. This contains an up to date listing of REMS™ drugs and the levels of risk mitigation required for each.

Table F-1
A sampling of Approved Products with REMS™

Drug Products	Levels of Risk Mitigation Required [1]			
	MG	CP	ETASU	IS
Actemra (tocilizumab) Injection		X		
Adasuve (loxapine) Inhalation Powder		X	X	X
Ampyra (dalfampridine) Extended-Release Tablets		X	X	X
Androgel (testosterone) 1% Gel		X		
Androgel (testosterone) 1.62% Gel	X			
Aranesp (darbepoetin alfa) Injection	X	X	X	X
Axiron (testosterone) Topical Solution	X			
Axiron (testosterone) Topical Solution				
Brilinta (ticagrelor) Tablets	X	X		
Bydureon (exenatide) Extended-Release for Injectable Suspension		X		
Caprelsa (vandetanib) Tablets	X	X	X	X
Chantix (varenicline) Tablets	X			
Eliquis (apixaban) Tablets		X		
Entereg (alvimopan) Capsules		X	X	X
Epogen/Procrit (epoetin alfa) Injection	X	X	X	X

Drug Products	Levels of Risk Mitigation Required [1]			
	MG	CP	ETASU	IS
Extraneal (icodextrin) Intraperitoneal Solution	X		X	X
Forteo (teriparatide [rDNA origin]) Injection	X	X		
Fortesta (testosterone) Gel	X			
Gattex (teduglutide [rDNA origin]) Injection		X	X	
Gilenya (fingolimod) Capsules		X		
H.P. Acthar Gel (repository corticotropin) Injection	X			
Juxtapid (lomitapide) Capsules			X	X
Krystexxa (pegloticase) Injection		X		
Kynamro (mipomersen sodium)			X	X
Letairis (ambrisentan) Tablets	X		X	X
Lotronex (alosetron hydrochloride) Tablets	X		X	X
Lumizyme (alglucosidase alfa)		X	X	X
Metoclopramide Oral Solution	X			
Metoclopramide Oral Solution	X			
Metoclopramide Oral Solution	X			
Mifeprex (mifepristone) Tablets	X		X	X
Multaq (dronedarone) Tablets	X	X		
Nplate (romiplostim) for Subcutaneous Injection		X		
Nulojix (belatacept)	X	X		
Omontys (peginesatide) Injection		X		
Pomalyst (pomalidomide) Capsules			X	X
Potiga (ezogabine) Tablets		X		
Prolia (denosumab) Injection	X	X		
Promacta (eltrombopag) Tablets		X		
Qsymia (phentermine and topiramate) Extended-Release Capsules	X		X	X
Revlimid (lenalidomide) Capsules			X	X
Sabril (vigabatrin) Oral Solution	X	X	X	X
Sabril (vigabatrin) Tablets	X	X	X	X
Soliris (eculizumab) Injection	X		X	

Drug Products	Levels of Risk Mitigation Required [1]			
	MG	CP	ETASU	IS
Stelara (ustekinumab) Injection		X		
Suboxone (buprenorphine and naloxone) Sublingual Film	X		X	X
Suboxone (buprenorphine and naloxone) Sublingual Tablets	X		X	X
Subutex (buprenorphine) Sublingual Tablets	X		X	X
Tapentadol Tablets	X			
Testim (testosterone) Gel	X			
Testosterone Gel	X			
Thalomid (thalidomide) Capsules			X	X
Tikosyn (dofetilide) Capsules	X		X	X
Tracleer (bosentan) Tablets	X		X	X
Truvada (emtricitabine and tenofovir disoproxil fumarate) Tablets	X		X	
Tysabri (natalizumab) Intravenous Injection	X		X	X
Versacloz (clozapine) Oral Suspension			X	X
Vibativ (telavancin) Injection	X	X		
Victoza (liraglutide) Injection		X		
Vivitrol (naltrexone) Extended-Release Injectable Suspension	X			
Xarelto (rivaroxaban) Tablets		X		
Xeljanz (tofacitinib) Tablets	X	X		
Xenazine (tetrabenazine) Tablets		X		
Xiaflex (collagenase clostridium histolyticum) Injection		X		
Yervoy (ipilimumab) Injection		X		
Zyban (bupropion hydrochloride) Sustained-Release Tablets	X			
Zyprexa Relprevv (olanzapine) Extended-Release Injection	X	X	X	X

[1] Column Guide
MG - Medication Guide
CP - Communication Plan
ETASU - Elements to Assure Safe Use
IS - Implementation System

The following are summaries of some common drugs that have restricted access programs:

THALOMID REMS™ Program

Thalidomide is a drug that has historically been associated with causing serious teratogenic malformations and, as a result, was removed from the market in the early 1960's.

Because of new therapeutic indications for thalidomide, the manufacturer reintroduced the drug onto the market. This company (Celgene) developed the THALOMID REMS™ program (formerly known as the S.T.E.P.S.® program) to reduce the likelihood of fetal exposure to the drug. Among the elements of this system are:

Prescriber Requirements

- The prescriber must enroll and becomes certified with Celgene for the THALOMID REMS™ program.
- The prescriber must counsel patient as to the benefits and risks of THALOMID.
- The prescriber must provide contraception and emergency contraception counseling.
- The prescriber must verify a negative pregnancy test for all female patients of reproductive potential.
- The prescriber must complete a THALOMID® (thalidomide) Patient-Physician Agreement Form with each patient and sends to the manufacturer (Celgene).
- The prescriber and patient must complete an applicable mandatory confidential survey.
- The prescriber must obtain an authorization number from Celgene and write it on every prescription.

- The prescriber must not prescribe more than a 4-week (28-day) supply, with no automatic refills or telephone prescriptions.
- The prescriber must send the THALOMID prescription to a certified pharmacy.

Pharmacy Requirements

- The pharmacy must be certified by Celgene for the THALOMID REMS™ program.
- The certified pharmacy must obtain a confirmation number from Celgene before dispensing.
- The certified pharmacy must dispense THALOMID to the patient along with a Medication Guide.

Rosiglitazone REMS™ Program

The following are the major elements of the Rosiglitazone REMS™ Program:

- A Medication Guide must be dispensed with each rosiglitazone prescription.
- Healthcare providers who prescribe rosiglitazone-containing medicines for outpatient or long-term care use must be certified by the manufacturer.
- Rosiglitazone may be dispensed only by specially certified pharmacies.
- Rosiglitazone may only be dispensed to patients who are enrolled in the Program.
- The manufacturer (GlaxoSmithKline) must submit REMS™ assessments to the FDA 6 months, 12 months, and annually from the date of initial approval of the Program.

The iPLEDGE Program for Isotretinoin

The iPLEDGE Program is a mandatory risk management program that was developed because of the danger of severe birth defects from the use of isotretinoin. The Program requires both male and female patients to enroll in a computerized registry in order to receive an isotretinoin product. Prescribers are also required to register to prescribe the drug while pharmacies and wholesalers must be registered in order for drug manufacturers to ship them the drug.

This program requires patients to sign a Patient Information/Informed Consent form informing them of the risks, including the possibility of depression or suicidal thoughts. They must also agree to monthly doctor visits for refills and agree not to share the medication with others. The doctor then registers each patient into the iPLEDGE database and gives them a special identifying code number. The pharmacist must check the database before filling an isotretinoin prescription to ensure that the patient is registered and has followed the rules.

Pharmacists should inform patients that infants may suffer severe brain and heart defects or mental retardation if even only a small dose of isotretinoin is taken by the parent, even for a brief period during pregnancy. The risk continues for 30 days after discontinuing the drug. A female patient must have the isotretinoin prescription filled within seven days of a pregnancy test that has confirmed that she is not pregnant.

REMS™ Program for LOTRONEX (alosetron hydrochloride)

The following are the important elements of the Lotronex REMS™ program:

- A Medication Guide must be dispensed with each LOTRONEX prescription.
- Health care providers who prescribe LOTRONEX must be certified in the Prescribing Program for LOTRONEX (PPL) and submit a Prescriber Enrollment Form (PEF) in which they

attest that they understand the proper use of the drug and the appropriate treatment of patients with LOTRONEX.

- Each patient who is prescribed LOTRONEX must sign a Patient Acknowledgement Form in which they attest the fact that they understand the uses and dangers of using LOTRONEX.
- The pharmacist may only fill LOTRONEX prescriptions if they have a PPL sticker on them.
- The manufacturer must file reports with the FDA every six months during the first year in the program and then annually in the following years.

As part of this program prescribers must affix Program stickers onto all prescriptions written for the drug. The drug must be dispensed with a Medication Guide for the patient. Telephoned, faxed or electronic prescriptions for Lotronex are not permitted under this Program. Prescriptions for Lotronex must be dispensed in its original package, which includes a Medication Guide, a package insert, and a follow-up survey enrollment form for patients.

Similar REMS™ programs are available for:

- Bosentan (Tracleer)
- Clozapine (Clozaril)
- Dofetilide (Tikosyn)
- Alendronate (Fosamax)

and other drug products listed in Table F-2.

Other Restricted Access REM™ Programs

Table F-2
Other Limited Access REM™ Programs

Drug Product	Limited Access Program	Elements of Program
Buprenorphine Transdermal (Butrans)	Butrans REMS™ Education Program	Prescriber must be enrolled
Epoetin alpha (Epogen, Procrit) and Darbepoetin (Aranesp)	ESA APPRISE Oncology Program	Prescriber and hospital must be enrolled Patient must sign a form indicating understanding of risk
Fentanyl buccal, nasal and transmucosal products.	A variety of programs	Distribution only permitted through authorized distributors
Hydromorphone ER (Exalgo)	Exalgo REMS™ Education Program	Prescriber must be enrolled
Mifepristone (Mifeprex)		Prescriber must be enrolled Limited distribution to office, clinic, or hospital
Oxycodone CR (Oxycontin)	Oxycontin REMS™ Educational Program	Prescriber must be enrolled

Off-label Uses of Drugs

After a drug product has been introduced onto the market, health professionals may find new therapeutic indications for it that are not included in the drug's product insert. The terms, "off-label" or "unlisted" uses, are sometimes used to describe such indications.

Although discouraged by the FDA, prescribers may prescribe the drug for these unofficial indications and pharmacists, using their professional discretion, may dispense such prescriptions. The drug manufacturer may not advertise such uses nor allow its sales representatives to detail such unofficial uses. However, the manufacturer may distribute peer-reviewed research papers that describe the off-label use of such drug products. There are several reference sources, including the *AHFS Drug Information*, which describe potential unlabeled drug indications.

Unit-dose Packaging and Labeling

Many pharmaceutical manufacturers provide their products, especially oral solid dosage forms such as capsules and tablets, in unit-dose packages. These strip packages are convenient for hospital use when daily supplies of the drug for individual patients are sent from the pharmacy to the nursing floors. Because of the small size of these packages, the FDA has issued guidelines as to what information should be on each unit-dose package. This information includes:

- Generic name and trade name, if appropriate.
- Quantity of active drug or drugs present (and the number of dosage units, if more than one).
- Name of the manufacturer, packer, or distributor.
- The repackager's lot number.
- The expiration date.
- Any other appropriate information concerning the specific drug (e.g. special storage requirements).

Many institutions, especially hospitals, repackage drug products into single dose units. A new expiration date must be provided for the repackaged product since the drug product has been transferred from the manufacturer's container, upon which its original expiration date was provided. Calculations for an appropriate expiration date will be considered later.

The return of unused unit-dose packages to the pharmacy for future dispensing is another issue that must be considered. Most states have established their own regulations. Some allow the return of unit dose packages only if originally dispensed to patients within the hospital setting or, in some cases, by a community pharmacy to a nursing home.

The expiration date requirement for a repackaged unit-dose package is fairly strict. While individual state guidelines may vary, the *USP/NF* states: "in the absence of stability data to the contrary, the expiration date should not exceed 25% of the remaining time between the date of repackaging and the original expiration date OR a 12 month dating from the date the drug was repackaged, whichever of these two is the LEAST."

> **Note**
>
> The above requirement is stricter than the general requirement in the *USP/NF* that multiple-unit containers have an expiration date not longer than the expiration date or one year from the date dispensed, whichever is less.

In an attempt to reduce medication errors, the FDA requires pharmaceutical companies to bar code all drug products supplied to hospitals. However, this requirement does not force individual hospitals to utilize bar codes. The ruling applies to prescription, biological, and nonprescription drug products, but not to physician samples. It also applies to single unit containers used in hospital unit-dose drug distribution systems. A bar code consists of a combination of bars and spaces with varying widths that allow encoding of pertinent information concerning a drug product. A scanner is employed in reading the bar code.

Rather than including the drug name, strength or manufacturer, the bar code must contain a drug's NDC. The pharmaceutical manufacturer may include other information that it considers appropriate. While not required, it has been suggested that the drug product's expiration date and lot release number be included.

The Uniform Code Council (UCC) has developed product bar code identification standards for manufacturing and retail industries. The bar code is considered by the FDA to be a part of the drug product label and is, therefore, subject to good manufacturing practices (GMP). Problems with bar code scanning may be reported to the FDA's Drug Quality Reporting System.

Customized Patient Med Paks

With the consent of the patient, the patient's caregiver, or the prescriber, some pharmacies are providing a customized patient medication package (Med Pak). This package may contain several solid oral dosage forms with directions that specifically indicate the day and time or period of time that the contents of each container are to be taken. The usual information for unit dose packages is required, plus a serial number for the patient Med Pak in addition to the prescription serial numbers for each drug product.

The expiration dating for the Med Pak is based upon the "beyond-use" dating principle but should not exceed 60 days from the date that the Med Pak was prepared.

The MedWatch Program

MedWatch, the FDA Medical Products Reporting Program, is an initiative designed to

- educate all health professionals about the critical importance of being aware of, monitoring for, and reporting adverse events and problems to the FDA and/or the manufacturer.

- ensure that new safety information is rapidly communicated to the medical community, thereby improving patient care.

The purpose of the MedWatch program is to enhance the effectiveness of post-marketing surveillance of medical products as they are used in clinical practice and to rapidly identify significant health hazards associated with these products.

The MedWatch program has four goals:

- To increase awareness of drug- and device-induced disease.
- To clarify what should (and should not) be reported to the agency.
- To simplify problem reporting by operating a single system for health professionals to report adverse events and product problems to the agency.
- To provide regular feedback to the health care community about safety issues involving medical products.

Health professionals may report serious adverse events and product problems with all medical products to MedWatch by mail, phone, fax, or over the Internet. A sample of the MedWatch Voluntary reporting form (Form FDA 3500) is depicted in Figure F-1 next page. Form FDA 3500B is a consumer friendly version of Form 3500 and Form FDA 3500A is a mandatory reporting form for IND reporters, manufacturers, distributors, importers, and user facility personnel.

S. Department of Health and Human Services

MEDWATCH

he FDA Safety Information and
dverse Event Reporting Program

For VOLUNTARY reporting of adverse events, product problems and product use errors

Page 1 of 3

Form Approved: OMB No. 0910-0291, Expires: 9/30/201
See PRA statement on revers

FDA USE ONLY

Triage unit sequence #

FDA Rec. Date

ote: For date prompts of "dd-mmm-yyyy" please use 2-digit day, 3-letter month bbreviation, and 4-digit year; for example, 01-Jul-2015.

A. PATIENT INFORMATION

. Patient Identifier — In Confidence

2. Age ☐ Year(s) ☐ Month(s) ☐ Week(s) ☐ Days(s)
or Date of Birth (*e.g., 08 Feb 1925*)

3. Sex ☐ Female ☐ Male

4. Weight ☐ lb ☐ kg

.a. Ethnicity (*Check ingle best answer*)
☐ Hispanic/Latino
☐ Not Hispanic/Latino

6.b. Race (*Check all that apply*)
☐ Asian ☐ American Indian or Alaskan Native
☐ Black or African American ☐ White
☐ Native Hawaiian or Other Pacific Islander

B. ADVERSE EVENT, PRODUCT PROBLEM

Check all that apply
☐ Adverse Event ☐ Product Problem (*e.g., defects/malfunctions*)
☐ Product Use Error ☐ Problem with Different Manufacturer of Same Medicine

Outcome Attributed to Adverse Event (*Check all that apply*)
☐ Death *Include date (dd-mmm-yyyy):*
☐ Life-threatening ☐ Disability or Permanent Damage
☐ Hospitalization – initial or prolonged ☐ Congenital Anomaly/Birth Defects
☐ Other Serious (Important Medical Events)
☐ Required Intervention to Prevent Permanent Impairment/Damage (Devices)

Date of Event (*dd-mmm-yyyy*)

4. Date of this Report (*dd-mmm-yyyy*)

Describe Event, Problem or Product Use Error

(Continue on page 3)

Relevant Tests/Laboratory Data, Including Dates

(Continue on page 3)

Other Relevant History, Including Preexisting Medical Conditions (*e.g., allergies, pregnancy, smoking and alcohol use, liver/kidney problems, etc.*)

(Continue on page 3)

C. PRODUCT AVAILABILITY

Product Available for Evaluation? (*Do not send product to FDA*)
☐ Yes ☐ No ☐ Returned to Manufacturer on (*dd-mmm-yyyy*)

D. SUSPECT PRODUCTS

Name, Manufacturer/Compounder, Strength (*from product label*)

– Name and Strength	#1 – NDC # or Unique ID
– Manufacturer/Compounder	#1 – Lot #
2 – Name and Strength	#2 – NDC # or Unique ID
2 – Manufacturer/Compounder	#2 – Lot #

3. Dose or Amount / Frequency / Route
#1
#2

4. Dates of Use (*From/To for each*) (*If unknown, give duration, or best estimate*) (*dd-mmm-yyyy*)
#1
#2

5. Diagnosis or Reason for Use (*indication*)
#1
#2

6. Is the Product Compounded?
#1 ☐ Yes ☐ No
#2 ☐ Yes ☐ No

7. Is the Product Over-the-Counter?
#1 ☐ Yes ☐ No
#2 ☐ Yes ☐ No

8. Expiration Date (*dd-mmm-yyyy*)
#1 #2

9. Event Abated After Use Stopped or Dose Reduced?
#1 ☐ Yes ☐ No ☐ Doesn't apply
#2 ☐ Yes ☐ No ☐ Doesn't apply

10. Event Reappeared After Reintroduction?
#1 ☐ Yes ☐ No ☐ Doesn't apply
#2 ☐ Yes ☐ No ☐ Doesn't apply

E. SUSPECT MEDICAL DEVICE

1. Brand Name

2. Common Device Name

2b. Procode

3. Manufacturer Name, City and State

4. Model # — Lot #
Catalog # — Expiration Date (*dd-mmm-yyyy*)
Serial # — Unique Identifier (UDI) #

5. Operator of Device
☐ Health Professional
☐ Lay User/Patient
☐ Other

6. If Implanted, Give Date (*dd-mmm-yyyy*)

7. If Explanted, Give Date (*dd-mmm-yyyy*)

8. Is this a single-use device that was reprocessed and reused on a patient? ☐ Yes ☐ No

9. If Yes to Item 8, Enter Name and Address of Reprocessor

F. OTHER (CONCOMITANT) MEDICAL PRODUCTS

Product names and therapy dates (*Exclude treatment of event*)

(Continue on page 3)

G. REPORTER (*See confidentiality section on back*)

1. Name and Address
Last Name: First Name:
Address:
City: State/Province/Region:
Country: ZIP/Postal Code:
Phone #: Email:

2. Health Professional? ☐ Yes ☐ No

3. Occupation

4. Also Reported to:
☐ Manufacturer/Compounder
☐ User Facility
☐ Distributor/Importer

5. If you do NOT want your identity disclosed to the manufacturer, please mark this box: ☐

ORM FDA 3500 (10/15) Submission of a report does not constitute an admission that medical personnel or the product caused or contributed to the event.

Figure F-1 - MedWatch Voluntary Reporting Form

Other Product Reporting Initiatives

Other initiatives exist for health professionals and consumers to report problems with drugs and medical devices. These include the following:

MedMARx™

This reporting system was developed by the USP to allow hospitals to anonymously report, track, and benchmark medication error data. It was developed to help reduce medication errors locally and nationally by permitting users to learn from the adverse experiences of others and share the successful solutions and policies that have been instituted.

Medical Device Problems

Health care facilities (e.g., hospitals, nursing homes, etc.), first under the Safe Medical Device Act of 1990 (SMDA) and then by the FDA Modernization Act of 1997, are legally required to report suspected medical device related deaths to both the FDA and the manufacturer, if known. Serious injuries must be reported to the manufacturer, or to the FDA if the manufacturer is unknown. Health professionals within a health care facility should familiarize themselves with their institution's procedures for reporting problems with medical devices.

Vaccine Problems

Adverse events and product problems that occur with vaccines should NOT be reported to the MedWatch program or on the MedWatch form but should be sent to the joint FDA/CDC Vaccine Adverse Event Reporting System (VAERS).

Veterinary Product Problems

Adverse events and product problems that occur with the use of medical products (drugs and devices) in animals should be reported to FDA's Center for Veterinary Medicine at 1-888-FDA-VETS (1-888-332-8387).

Drug Recalls

If a marketed drug product exhibits problems, the manufacturer is encouraged to issue a drug recall notice. Problems may vary from minor issues with a particular manufacturing lot to serious drug-related adverse effects such as a high incidence of hepatotoxicity. Drug recalls are divided into three classes.

- **Class I** - The drug product may cause serious, adverse health consequences including death. The recall should include stocks located in pharmacies and notification of patients to whom the drug has been dispensed.
- **Class II** - The drug product may cause temporary or reversible effects but the probability of serious adverse effects is remote. The recall will usually include stocks located in pharmacies.
- **Class III** - The drug product is unlikely to cause any adverse health consequence.

It is the manufacturer's responsibility to send written recall notices to all wholesalers and pharmacies for recalls in the Class I and II categories. There may be some Class III recalls that are handled with written notices as well.

It is the pharmacist's responsibility to be aware of all recalls either received in the mail or read in the pharmaceutical literature.

Occasionally, an ingredient present in either a prescription or nonprescription drug product is determined to be potentially dangerous. The FDA may request that a manufacturer of a certain product discontinue sales and/or remove the product from the market. This request for a "voluntary" discontinuation or removal is invariably honored. An example of this action was the FDA's request that all companies discontinue marketing products containing phenylpropanolamine (PPA). This was done subsequent to the issuance, by the FDA, of a public health advisory concerning the risk of hemorrhagic stroke or bleeding into the brain linked to the use of PPA.

Prescription Compounding vs. Manufacturing

With the advent of a multitude of commercial prescription drug products, the pharmaceutical industry has relieved the pharmacist of the need for most prescription compounding. The inherent right of the pharmacist to compound prescriptions has been challenged in recent years primarily because of several unfortunate instances in which pharmacists extended their practice into the area of manufacturing. Recently, further attention has been drawn to this issue because of a number of reported bacterial or fungal contaminations of parenteral products apparently compounded by compounding pharmacies and then distributed throughout the U.S.

The critical issue is: When does small-scale prescription compounding become manufacturing? The FDA Compliance Policy Guide of 1992 states that pharmacies may compound drugs extemporaneously if:

- the quantity prepared is reasonable for filling either existing prescriptions or those anticipated based upon prescribing habits of local prescribers and/or prescriptions already on file.
- the dosage forms prepared are not being compounded, provided, or sold to other pharmacies or third parties such as physician's offices.
- the drug products compounded are not ones already available from commercial sources. That is, they are not compounded versions of FDA-approved drug products.
- the ingredients included in a compounded dosage form meet official standards, usually those found in the *USP/NF*. If an ingredient does not have an official monograph, it may be used to compound a prescription if it is a component of or an approved drug product, or it is on a list of approved substances developed by the Secretary of the U.S. Department of Health and Human Services.
- the pharmacy does not actively solicit business for specific compounded drug products by advertising or by otherwise

promoting their compounding capabilities. However, the pharmacy may advertise to both the public and health professionals that it specializes in prescription compounding. The 1997 FDA Modernization Act included a provision that states that compounding pharmacies are not manufacturers and are therefore exempt from standard FDA regulation on that basis. The Act prohibits pharmacists from advertising or promoting compounded drugs. In 2002, the U.S. Supreme Court modified this policy by ruling that the FDA could not restrict pharmacists from advertising or promoting products solely because they were compounded.

- the pharmacy does not attempt to compound a drug product which is on the list of products that have been withdrawn or removed from the market because they were unsafe or ineffective.
- the pharmacy limits its interstate distribution of compounded products to not more than 5% of the total prescriptions filled by that pharmacy.

May a pharmacist develop a sustained-release drug product similar to a commercial product under his/her prerogative as a compounding pharmacist? The answer is no. This activity is not permissible because a compounding pharmacist is not allowed to compound drug products that are commercially available. In addition, preparing a quantity of the compounded product would probably place the operation into the classification of manufacturing, not compounding.

2013 Drug Quality and Security Act

As a result of numerous deaths caused by contaminated parenteral steroid products manufactured by New England Compounding Center, Congress passed the 2013 Drug Quality and Security Act. This legislation permits compounding pharmacies to register with the FDA as "outsourcing facilities" and to be subject to rules dealing with quality control and oversight that are similar to rules that apply to large drug manufacturers.

However, there is no requirement for compounding pharmacies to register with the FDA nor any FDA-specified procedures that must be followed to ensure safety. Some compounding pharmacies do register with the FDA. However, just because a pharmacy is "FDA-registered" does not mean it is routinely inspected by the FDA nor that the FDA has reviewed or approved any compounded preparations. A pharmacy claiming to be "FDA approved" is misleading and inaccurate.

Expiration Dating for Compounded Prescriptions

The pharmacist should base expiration dating or beyond-use dating upon the stability information available. In the absence of stability information, the following guidelines are appropriate for beyond-use dating.

- For nonaqueous liquids and solids made using commercially manufactured products: not more than 25% of the time remaining on the commercial product or a maximum of six months, whichever is less.
- For aqueous solutions made from solids obtained from commercially manufactured drug products: 14 days when stored at a cold temperature.
- For all others: for the duration of therapy, but not more than 30 days.

> ### Note
>
> Compounded radiopharmaceuticals and Positron Emission Tomography (P.E.T.) drugs are exempt from these compounding standards.

Compounding of Sterile Products for Use in the Home

The *USP/NF* has issued guidelines for the preparation by pharmacies of sterile drug products intended for dispensing to patients in home settings. These products are designated as "home-use sterile drug products" or "HSD's". The HSD is typically delivered to a residence, which is not equipped with a sterile preparation area, and the administration is not under the direct supervision of the dispensing pharmacist.

Such extemporaneously prepared injectable and ophthalmic drug products must be compounded in a strictly defined environment to assure sterility and safety. Techniques required to prepare such products are classified as "low–risk" or "high-risk" mainly based upon the types of ingredients to be used, dosage forms to be prepared, and the aseptic techniques required.

Low-Risk

These are techniques involving commercially available sterile products that are manufactured in a "closed system". Examples include:

- Transfer of a solution from a commercial vial or ampule with a needle and syringe.
- Compounding total parenteral nutrition (TPN) solutions using commercially available sterile solutions.
- Transfer of sterile solutions into elastomeric devices.

High-Risk

These are techniques involving more complex skills to assure sterility and safety of the final product. They are further classified into two categories.

Category I activities include the following techniques:

- Pooling sterile drug products for subsequent transfers.
- Complex compounding involving numerous aseptic processes.

- Preparing an infusion intended for multi-day use in a portable pump or reservoir system.

An example of a Category I compounding activity would be the preparation of TPN's using automated compounding devices.

Category II activities involve ingredients, products, and techniques which pose the greatest risk of contamination. In most instances, the final product will have to be sterilized by the compounder. Examples include:

- Using non-sterile drug substances in preparing a product.
- Using "open systems" such as the compounding of morphine solutions for injection or infusion using morphine powder.
- Compounding sterile nutritional solutions using non-sterile ingredients during which the initial mixing is performed in an unsealed or nonsterile reservoir.

Sample Questions

1. Which of the following actions is (are) permissible under the FDA rules for prescription compounding by pharmacies?

   I. Informing an allergy specialist that the pharmacy can economically compound 50 mg diphenhydramine capsules.

   II. Sending brochures to nurse practitioners that indicate that the pharmacy compounds topical ointments for the treatment of skin rashes.

   III. Advertising to ophthalmologists that the pharmacy can compound sterile, isotonic ophthalmic solutions.

   (A) I only (B) III only (C) I & II only

   (D) II & III only (E) I, II, & III

2. A pharmacy begins to receive prescriptions for a capsule mixture that is not available commercially. The usual prescription is for a total of 14 capsules with two refills and the patient is to take one capsule daily. What is the maximum number of capsules the pharmacist may compound under FDA guidelines?

(A) 14 only

(B) 28 only

(C) 42 only

(D) Not more than 100

(E) A sufficient quantity to meet anticipated prescriptions and refills

3. Which of the following actions may a pharmacy specializing in extemporaneous compounding undertake?

I. Advertise and promote its compounding services with a brochure.

II. Describe its capabilities to prepare sterile parenteral admixtures.

III. Describe dollar savings to customers of a compounded pilocarpine 2% ophthalmic solution.

(A) I only (B) III only (C) I & II only

(D) II & III only (E) I, II, & III

4. A pharmaceutical manufacturer includes a color additive, that is not FDA approved, in a topical cream formulation. The product could be removed from the market as being:

(A) misbranded (B) contaminated

(C) improperly labeled (D) adulterated

(E) hyperallergenic

5. The number of categories of drug recalls is ___?___ with recall number ___?___ the most serious.

(A) 4 and 1 (B) 3 and 3 (C) 3 and 1

(D) 4 and 4 (E) 5 and 1

6. Which of the following techniques would be classified as "low-risk" for pharmacists to perform based upon USP guidelines for preparation of home-use sterile drug products?

   I. Placing 20 mEq of Potassium Chloride Injection into a one liter bag of Sterile D5W using a needle and syringe.

   II. Mixing 500 mL of a Sterile Amino Acids 5% Solution with 500 mL of D50W by gravity flow.

   III. Aseptically transferring 20 mL of Sterile Morphine Sulfate Injection into a 50 mL elastomeric device.

   (A) I only (B) III only (C) I & II only
   (D) II & III only (E) I, II, & III

7. Which of the following techniques would be classified as "high-risk, Category II" for pharmacists to perform based upon USP guidelines for preparation of home-use sterile drug products?

   I. Compounding an injection solution using nonsterile drug powder and then passing the solution through a 0.22 micron filter.

   II. Mixing several sterile solutions together to make a batch of TPN injections.

   III. Pooling several vials of a chemotherapeutic drug injection for subsequent subdivision into individual minibags.

   (A) I only (B) III only (C) I & II only
   (D) II & III only (E) I, II, & III

8. The designation of "off-label" for a drug indicates which of the following?

   (A) Therapeutic use not approved by the FDA.
   (B) Therapeutic use that is listed on the drug product's label but not found in the product insert.
   (C) Formerly approved drug product recently withdrawn from the market.
   (D) A former therapeutic use of a drug, which is no longer recognized.
   (E) A therapeutic use suggested by the manufacturer on TV but not included in the product insert.

9. A prescriber writes a prescription for a drug product and specifies a use that is not recognized as an indication for the drug in the product insert. Which of the following actions is most appropriate?

   (A) Fill the prescription.
   (B) Fill the prescription but inform the patient that it is not for an appropriate use.
   (C) Inform the prescriber that it is illegal to write such a prescription.
   (D) Request that the prescriber write on the prescription face the term "off-label use".
   (E) Refuse to fill the prescription since it is illegal to do so.

10. A community pharmacy that describes itself as being "FDA Approved" for compounding:

   (A) must be inspected yearly by the FDA
   (B) must have completed an FDA approved program for compounding
   (C) must be supervised by pharmacist with a PharmD degree
   (D) has a misleading and inaccurate description
   (E) can manufacture products for foreign consumption.

Answers:

(1) D (2) E (3) C (4) D (5) C (6) E
(7) A (8) A (9) A (10) D

Section G

Filling and Dispensing Prescriptions

Whenever the pharmacist encounters a prescription or medication order for a specific drug product, one of his/her first considerations should be whether the drug is classified as a non-controlled prescription drug or as a controlled substance. Most controlled substance regulations are stricter than those for other drug products, particularly with respect to inventory and labeling requirements, and limits on quantities that may be dispensed.

Controlled substance regulations will be covered in great detail in Section H of this Guide. In this section, the general regulations for the filling and dispensing of prescriptions will be considered, i.e. rules that apply to almost all prescription products.

Federal vs. State Regulations

Federal and individual state pharmacy laws sometimes differ. In such instances, the more strict regulation usually predominates and must be followed.

> ### *Note*
>
> The individuals responsible for the MPJE® are careful to avoid questions that fall into the "gray area" i.e., those questions concerning areas of pharmacy practice which either have conflicts between federal and state law or involve issues that have not yet been clearly resolved.
>
> Before a question is accepted as a test item, its worthiness is evaluated by being tested as a sample question on other examinations. As explained previously, always choose the stricter law or regulation when there is a conflict between federal and state law. The following guidelines may be helpful when answering MPJE® questions.

Authorization to Prescribe

Each state specifies those types of health professionals who may prescribe and sets prescribing limits on prescribers such as nurse practitioners, physician assistants, etc. Questions in this area are usually based on individual state laws.

Health Professionals That Self-Prescribe

Can a legitimate prescriber write a prescription for his/her own use? Self-prescribing is acceptable in most states, but some have prohibited the self-prescribing of controlled substances.

Pharmacist's Obligation to Fill a Prescription

A pharmacist may refuse to fill any prescription for any one of several "good" reasons including:

- The prescription is a suspected forgery or is fictitious. The difference between these two terms is mainly one of semantics. A forged prescription is one that has been written using the name and information of a legitimate prescriber. A fictitious prescription is one that someone has prepared by creating information based upon a nonexistent prescriber.
- The pharmacist would be violating a law if he/she fills the prescription.
- The drug or drug product is not in stock.
- The pharmacist believes that the drug product may be harmful to the patient.

Prescription Refills

One issue that faces every prescriber and pharmacist is whether a specific prescription may be refilled. Controlled substances have tighter limitations as to whether or how often a prescription may be refilled. To refill a prescription for other drugs, the prescriber must have indicated how many refills the patient is to have and/or a time limitation for refills to be obtained. Many states have established stricter limitations, usually a time span of not more than one year. All refills must be indicated on the back of the original prescription or by using another reliable recording system (e.g. a computer).

If a pharmacist receives a prescription for a nonprescription drug product with specific refill directions he/she is bound to the refill limits, particularly if the dose prescribed is greater than normal or if the drug is a Schedule V controlled substance.

Prescription Ownership

Once a prescription has been filled and dispensed, the prescription is legally owned by the pharmacy. It should not be removed from the files except by court order. If the prescriber or patient requests the actual prescription, the pharmacist should refuse but offer a copy of the prescription.

Prescription File Storage Period

Most states require prescription records to be kept for two to five years. The FDA claims that it may request records of drug distribution dating back five years. As of January 1, 2005 the Medicare Modernization Act of 2003 requires prescription records to be kept for ten years. Practically, most pharmacies keep prescription records indefinitely.

Prescription Container Labeling

In October 2012 the USP described new standards for universal approach to format, appearance, content and language of instructions for medicines in containers dispensed by pharmacists. These ultimately were published in USP 36–NF 31 (USP General Chapter <17>) and became official standards on May 1, 2013. Some of the important elements of these standards include the following:

1. The top of the prescription label should specify the patient's name, prescription (serial) number, the drug name (full generic and brand name), the strength, and clear directions for use provided in simple language.
2. Other less critical, but important content, such as prescription number, expiration date, quantity, physical description, etc. should not supercede critical patient information. Such less critical information should be placed in a less prominent place, e.g. at the bottom of the label.
3. The readability of the label should be improved by the use of familiar large fonts such as 12 point Times Roman or 11 point Arial.
4. Drug names should be spelled out rather than using an abbreviation or acronym (e.g. use "acetaminophen" rather than "APAP").

5. Explicit instructions must be clarified. For example,
   (a) Numbers should be used instead of alphabetic characters, i.e. "2" instead of "two"
   (b) Implicit directions such as "Take 2 tablets twice daily" should be avoided. Instead, explicit directions such as "Take 2 tablets in the morning and 2 tablets in the evening" are recommended.
   (c) specific hour designations, such as 8 AM and 10 PM or every 12 hours should be avoided. Instead, use "in the morning or after breakfast".
6. Unless the patient prefers that it not appear, the prescription label should include the purpose for use if it is included on the prescription. Use terms such as "for high blood pressure" rather than "for hypertension"
7. The pharmacist should address limited English proficiency. When possible, label directions should be in the patient's preferred language. However the drug name must also be in English to aid emergency personnel.
8. The pharmacy name, address, telephone number, etc should not supersede the above critical information and should be placed away from dosing instructions.
9. The prescription label should also include prescriber's name.
10. The date on the prescription label should indicate when the prescription was either written or dispensed. Some states require that the date of a refill be used when the prescription is refilled.
11. Inclusion of expiration dating, lot number of the drug product, and/or the name of the drug manufacturer is left to the discretion of individual states.

Enforcement of these labeling standards are at the discretion of individual state boards of pharmacy as are the USP standards for sterile and non sterile pharmaceutical compounding.

Tall Man Lettering

The concept of "Tall Man Lettering" has emerged as a means of reducing medication errors. It is based upon the use of larger (taller) letters in a drug name to make the drug name more easily distinguishable from drugs that have a similar spelling. In 2012, the FDA and the Institute for Safe Medication Practices (ISMP) published a list of recommended Tall Man letters for look-alike drugs including, but not limited to:

- acetaZOLAMIDE vs. acetoHEXAMIDE
- buPROPion vs. busPIRone
- chlorproMAZINE vs. chlorproPAMIDE
- clomiPHENE vs. clomiPRAMINE
- cycloSERINE vs. cycloSPORINE
- DAUNOrubicin vs. DOXOrubicin
- DOBUTamine vs. DOPamine
- hydrALAZINE vs. hydrOXYzine
- TOLAZamide vs. TOLBUTamide
- vinBLAStine vs. vinCRIStine

Expiration Dating vs. Beyond-Use Dating

While the term "expiration date" originated with the dating required on manufacturer's containers, the term "beyond-use date" is now used to describe the dating of drug products that are dispensed by pharmacists. The simplest example would be an antibiotic powder, which is reconstituted with purified water by the pharmacist.

The traditional "beyond-use" expiration date for the reconstituted antibiotic solution is typically ten days, even though the "expiration date" indicated on the manufacturer's container may be two years for the unreconstituted powder.

The USP has issued guidelines for dispensing pharmacists with regard to beyond-use dating. For oral solid dosage forms, the beyond-use date is somewhat arbitrary depending upon the pharmacist's professional judgment or specific state regulations. In all cases, the beyond-use date may not be greater than the expiration date on the manufacturer's original package. For dosage forms in multidose containers, i.e. drug products in prescription vials, the beyond-use date must be the shorter of either the manufacturer's expiration date or not more than one year from the date the drug is dispensed.

While regulations dealing with expiration dates for drug products dispensed by prescription are in the hands of the individual states, the FDA specifies that labels for drug products dispensed to nursing homes, intermediate care, and skilled nursing facilities must have beyond-use dating.

Questions concerning expiration dating must be answered carefully since there are several possible scenarios that involve expiration dating. These include:

- **Expiration dating for a commercial drug product as established by the manufacturer.**

  The manufacturer has established this dating for a specific package and a specific product. Most manufacturers indicate the expiration date on the container in terms of month and year. For example, the designation of July 2019 indicates that the manufacturer has data showing that the drug product will remain within *USP/NF* specifications at least through July 31, 2019. Homeopathic products are exempted from the requirement of an expiration dating.

- **Expiration dating for a unit dose package that has been prepared from a bulk container of a commercial drug**

product.

The repackager, usually a pharmacist who is supervising the operation, will determine this dating. The current guideline provided in the *USP/NF* is for repackaged drug products to have the shorter of two potential dates:

— 12 months maximum or

— 25% of the time remaining on the original package of bulk drug product

Many states, however, have established other guidelines by allowing longer dating - as much as one year maximum or 25% of the time remaining on the manufacturer's expiration date, whichever is less. Since the *USP* is presently reviewing its guidelines, it is unlikely that the MPJE® will have questions on expiration dating for unit-dose packages.

> **Study Tip**
>
> One possible question that could be asked is how the FDA and other inspection bodies classify a unit-dose product that does not have an expiration date? The answer is that the product is misbranded.

Sample Calculation

Assume that an original drug product had an expiration date of Sept 2018. A pharmacist repackages the product on January 1, 2018 and uses the FDA guidelines of six months maximum or 25% of the time remaining on the original package of bulk drug product.

A six-month maximum will produce a useful product life of January through June and will result in the expiration date of June 2018. The rule using 25% of time remaining will result in the calculation of 25% of the time from the date of repackaging to the manufacturer's expiration date (a total period of nine months). Twenty-five percent of nine months is 2.25 months, thereby yielding the expiration date of March 7, 2018.

In the above example the March date is shorter than the June date and must be used. Be careful! An answer of March 2018 would be incorrect since that implies an expiration date of March 31, 2018. If the choices of answers are (A) Jan 2018 (B) Feb 2018 (C) Mar 2018 (D) June 2018 (E) Sept 2018, you would have to select (B) as the correct choice. Hopefully the examiners will not be this tricky!

- **Expiration dating for individual prescriptions being dispensed by a pharmacist.**

  There is no federal law concerning this type of dating. Instead, some states have established their own guidelines, usually a maximum of one year.

- **Manufacturer's expiration dating.**

  All pharmaceuticals must have a clearly legible expiration date on the package. The manufacturer establishes the expiration date for a commercial drug product by conducting extensive stability testing of the drug dosage form in the final package. Data is submitted to the FDA to validate the dating, which is usually a time span of several years.

  Most manufacturers indicate the expiration date on the container labeling in terms of month and year. For example, the designation of July 2018 indicates that the manufacturer has data showing that the drug product will remain within *USP/NF* specifications at least through July 31, 2018. To be more specific, if the official standard for a 100 mg tablet is "not less than 95% of labeled claim", one would expect that on July 31st, the active amount of drug in the tablet would not be less than 95 mg.

  Pharmacists may not continue to dispense a drug product once its expiration date has passed. Most states require the pharmacist to remove any expired products from the working stock to a quarantine area until the product can either be destroyed or returned to the manufacturer.

Poison Prevention Packaging Act (PPPA)

In 1970 the federal government enacted the Poison Prevention Packaging Act (PPPA). Its purpose was to protect children less than five years of age from accidental poisoning. Under the supervision of the Consumer Product Safety Commission (CPSC) since 1973, the PPPA requires child-resistant closures that prevent access to almost all prescription drugs, nonprescription drugs, and hazardous household products in order to protect young children from serious injury or illness caused by their accidental ingestion. Among the drug products required to be packaged in such child-resistant packaging by the PPPA are

- **Aspirin** – all oral dosage forms
- **Methyl salicylate** – liquid products containing more than 5% by weight unless packaged in pressurized spray containers
- **Controlled substances** – all oral dosage forms
- **Prescription Drugs** – all oral dosage forms
- **Iron** – all non-injectable drug products and most iron-containing dietary supplements that contain 250 mg or more of elemental iron per package
- **Acetaminophen** – oral dosage forms containing more than one gram of acetaminophen per single package
- **Diphenhydramine** – oral dosage forms containing more than the equivalent of 66 mg of diphenhydramine base per package
- **Ibuprofen** – oral dosage forms that contain one gram or more of ibuprofen in a single package
- **Loperamide** – oral dosage forms containing more than 0.045mg of loperamide in a single package
- **Mouthwash** – Single packages that contain three grams or

more of ethanol

- **Lidocaine** – products that contain more than 5mg of lidocaine in a single package
- **Dibucaine** – products that contain more than 0.5mg of dibucaine in a single package
- **Naproxen** – oral dosage forms that contain 250mg or more of naproxen in a single package
- **Ketoprofen** – oral dosage forms that contain 50mg or more of ketoprofen in a single package
- **Fluoride** – products containing more than 50mg of elemental fluoride and 0.5% fluoride in a single package
- **Minoxidil** – products that contain more than 14mg of minoxidil in a single package
- **Nonprescription drugs** – oral products that contain any active ingredient that was previously available in oral form by prescription only

Some drug products are intended by the pharmaceutical manufacturer to be dispensed by the pharmacist in their original containers. Such units must also meet the requirements of the Poison Prevention Packaging Act (PPPA).

Other provisions of the PPPA include:

- If an OTC product is marketed in several sizes, one package size is not required to have a safety closure. Such products must include on their label the statement, "This package for households without young children."
- All new and refilled prescriptions must be dispensed in a child-resistant closure unless:
  - — the prescriber specifies that none is to be used. This may only be specified for each individual prescription, i.e. a physician cannot provide a blanket child-resistant waiver directive that applies to all of a patient's prescriptions.

— the patient indicates that they do not want such a closure. Patients may ask for a non-child-resistant container for a single prescription or they may provide a "blanket waiver" that directs the pharmacist to never provide a child-resistant container when their prescriptions are filled. In either case, it is advisable to have the patient sign a waiver on the back of each individual prescription and to reconfirm the patient's wishes on a regular basis.

> **Note**
>
> Prescribers may only provide a waiver for the use of a child-resistant container for a single prescription at a time. Patients, however, may provide a blanket waiver for the use of child-resistant containers for one or more of their prescriptions.

— the container is being used in a hospital or similar institution in which the drugs are maintained and administered by health professionals. However, child-resistant containers should be used by pharmacies providing drug products to nursing homes.

- When preparing prescription refills for patients, both parts (body and closure) of plastic container units must be replaced. If the container body is constructed of glass, it may be reused but the plastic closure must be replaced. This is a safety precaution since many plastic closures may lose their child-resistant features after repeated use. The pharmacy may employ reversible closures (those designed to be used as either safety or regular tops) although this practice is discouraged by the CPSC.

Since the enactment of the PPPA, a number of drug products have been exempted from the child-resistant packaging requirements by special request of the manufacturers. They include:

1. Sublingual dosage forms of nitroglycerin,

2. Sublingual and chewable forms of isosorbide dinitrate in dosage strengths of 10 milligrams or less.
3. Erythromycin ethylsuccinate granules for oral suspension and oral suspensions in packages containing not more than 8 grams or the equivalent of erythromycin.
4. Erythromycin ethylsuccinate tablets in packages containing no more than the equivalent of 16 grams erythromycin.
5. Anhydrous cholestyramine in powder form.
6. Potassium supplements in unit dose forms, including individually wrapped effervescent tablets, unit dose vials of liquid potassium, and powdered potassium in unit dose packets, containing not more than 50 milliequivalents per unit dose.
7. Sodium fluoride drug preparations, including liquid and tablet forms, containing no more than 264 milligrams of sodium fluoride per package.
8. Betamethasone tablets packaged in manufacturers' dispenser packages containing no more than 12.6 milligrams betamethasone.
9. Mebendazole in tablet form in packages containing not more than 600 milligrams of the drug.
10. Methylprednisolone in tablet form in packages containing not more than 84 milligrams of the drug.
11. Colestipol in powder form in packages containing not more than 5 grams of the drug.
12. Pancrelipase preparations in tablet, capsule, or powder form.
13. Cyclically administered oral contraceptives in mnemonic (memory-aid) dispenser packages which rely solely upon the activity of one or more progestogen or estrogen substances.
14. Prednisone in tablet form when dispensed in packages containing no more than 105 milligrams of the drug.
15. Conjugated estrogen tablets when dispensed in mnemonic

dispenser packages containing not more than 32.0 milligrams of the drug.

16. Norethindrone acetate tablets in mnemonic dispenser packages containing not more than 50 milligrams of the drug.
17. Medroxyprogesterone acetate tablets.
18. Sacrosidase (sucrase) preparations in a solution of glycerol and water.
19. Hormone Replacement Therapy products that rely solely upon the activity of one or more progestogen or estrogen substances.

The Consumer Product Safety Commission (CPSC), which has jurisdiction of the PPPA, has established the testing protocols for child-resistant packaging (CRP). Test panels used to assess such packaging generally consist of two groups:

- Children under five years of age.
- Adults 50 to 70 years of age.

A package will fail the child-resistant test if more than 20% of the children can open the package in a total of ten minutes. However, to meet adult-friendly requirements, 90% of a one hundred person adult panel must be able to open and close the package in five minutes; and then do so a second time within one minute.

Federal Anti-Tampering Act (1982)

Following several incidents of deliberate contamination of OTC products with poisonous substances, Congress enacted the Federal Anti-Tampering Act in 1982. Provisions of this Act require that tamper-evident packaging be used for select OTC products and cosmetics, particularly those taken orally. The package may feature an indicator or barrier to limit access. If disturbed, some visible evidence of entry will be evident. For example, a simple plastic film seal or a tab around the container closure is sufficient. The product label must indicate that it is a tamper-evident package and should indicate how a consumer can determine if the package has been tampered with.

> ### Note
>
> In reviewing this chapter, remember that the tamper-evident and the poison prevention regulations are different.

Sample Questions

1. Enforcement of the PPPA is basically under the jurisdiction of thc:

   (A) Consumer Product Safety Commission (CPSC)

   (B) Federal Trade Commission (FTC)

   (C) Food and Drug Administration (FDA)

   (D) Federal Alcohol, Tobacco and Firearms Agency

   (E) Health Care Financing Administration (HCFA)

2. Permission to not use a poison prevention closure on a prescription may be granted by the

   I. patient

   II. prescriber

   III. pharmacist

   (A) I only (B) III only (C) I & II only

   (D) II & III only (E) I, II, & III

3. The Poison Prevention Packaging Act (PPPA) was intended to protect

   I. young children

   II. geriatric patients

   III. visually impaired patients

(A) I only (B) III only (C) I & II only
(D) II & III only (E) I, II, & III

4. When refilling a prescription that requires a poison prevention container, the pharmacist must always replace a

   I. plastic closure
   II. plastic container
   III. glass container

   (A) I only (B) III only (C) I & II only
   (D) II & III only (E) I, II, & III

5. Original packages of nitroglycerin, which are exempt from the requirements of the Poison Prevention Packaging Act, include:

   I. sublingual tablets
   II. ointments
   III. oral tablets

   (A) I only (B) III only (C) I & II only
   (D) II & III only (E) I, II, & III

6. In which of the following situations are child-resistant closures not required?

   I. When a prescriber dispenses a prescription drug directly from his/her office.
   II. When a hospital pharmacy fills a prescription for an outpatient.
   III. When a hospital pharmacy fills a prescription for an inpatient.

   (A) I only (B) III only (C) I & II only
   (D) II & III only (E) I, II, & III

7. Which of the following types of drug products are NOT required to be dispensed in a poison prevention package?

   (A) An analgesic for a child over the age of two.
   (B) An analgesic for a child over the age of five.
   (C) An analgesic for an adult.
   (D) A bronchodilator in a metered aerosol container.
   (E) Estrogen tablets for a female over the age of 65.

8. Which of the following OTC products must be packaged in a tamper-evident package?

   I. mouthwash
   II. contact lens solution
   III. insulin

   (A) I only (B) III only (C) I & II only
   (D) II & III only (E) I, II, & III

9. Which of the following products must be packaged with a child-resistant closure?

   I. A commercial container of 30 acetaminophen 325mg tablets.
   II. A commercial container of 10 ketoprofen (Actron) 12.5mg tablets.
   III. An aerosol topical product containing 2% methyl salicylate.

   (A) I only (B) III only (C) I & II only
   (D) II & III only (E) I, II, & III

Answers:

(1) A (2) C (3) A (4) C (5) C (6) B
(7) D (8) C (9) C

Patient Package Inserts (PPIs)

Many potentially dangerous drugs must be dispensed with a Patient Package Insert (PPI). This is a document, written in lay language, which is intended to educate the client about the proper use and potential dangers inherent in the use of the product accompanying the PPI. PPIs must be provided to patients receiving prescriptions for products such as Accutane, "statin" drugs, as well as to those receiving estrogen or progestin-containing products.

These rules apply to all physicians, community pharmacists, and hospital pharmacists who dispense drugs. It also means that hospital pharmacies must provide PPIs to hospitalized patients who are receiving estrogen and progestin-containing products such as Premarin, oral contraceptive products, and intrauterine contraceptive devices containing these drugs. This can done by providing patients with the PPI prior to administering the first dose of such drug products. Subsequent PPIs may be provided to the patient every thirty days thereafter. This PPI requirement also applies to patients in long term care facilities such as nursing homes.

Prescribers who dispense prescriptions from their offices are NOT exempt from the requirement of providing PPIs.

In January 2006, the FDA released a major revision to the PPI guidelines. The revision included a section called Highlights which summarizes the most important information about the benefits and risks of the drug product. It also required that the PPI have a Table of Contents and the date of initial product approval. It also requires that the PPI contain a toll-free phone number and Internet address to encourage more widespread reporting of information regarding adverse events.

Medication Guides (MedGuides)

As part of an initiative to provide patients with comprehensive information about drug products that have been prescribed for them, the FDA, in 1995, announced the Medication Guide (MedGuides) program. This program provides standards for the distribution and quality of written prescription information material or MedGuides to be dispensed to patients. Such guides would be prepared by drug manufacturers on a voluntary basis and in language easily understood by patients. The FDA requires MedGuides for products when:

- patient labeling could prevent serious adverse effects.
- the product has serious risks relative to benefits.
- patient adherence to directions is crucial.

The MedGuide paper sheets or the means to produce them (e.g. by providing PDF files suitable for printing in a pharmacy) are distributed by drug product manufacturers to dispensers, who are then required to provide them to patients.

Manufacturers must obtain FDA approval before distributing their MedGuides. There are currently several hundred drug products that must be dispensed with MedGuides. Some of these include:

- Advair Diskus (salmeterol & fluticasone)
- Anaprox (naproxen sodium)
- Avonex (interferon beta-1a)
- Concerta (methylphenidate)
- Cordarone (amiodarone)
- Coumadin (warfarin)
- Duragesic (fentanyl)
- Elidel Cream (pimecrolimus)
- Emsam (selegeline transdermal system)
- Epzicom (abacavir & lamivudine)
- Forteo (teriparatide)
- Infergen (interferon alfacon-1)
- Isotretinoin
- Lariam (mefloquine)
- Lexapro (escitalopram oxalate)
- Lindane shampoo and lotion

- Lotronex (alosetron)
- Mifeprex (mifepristone)
- Nolvadex (tamoxifen)
- NSAIDS
- Palladone (hydromorphone)
- Pegasys (peginterferon alfa-2a)
- PEG-Intron (pegylated interferon alfa-2b)
- Protopic Ointment (tacrolimus)
- Rebetol (ribavirin)
- Rebif (interferon beta-1a)
- Remicade (infliximab)
- Revlimid (lenlidomide)
- Ritalin (methylphenidate)
- Roferon-A (interferon alpha-2A)
- Serevent Diskus (salmeterol xinafoate)
- Soltamox (tamoxifen oral solution)
- Soriatane (acitretin)
- Strattera (atomoxetine)
- Symlin (pramlintide)
- Tracleer (bosentan)
- Trizivir (abacavir, lamivudine, & zidovudine)
- Viramune (nevirapine)
- Xolair (omalizumab)
- Xyrem (sodium oxybate)
- Ziagen (abacavir)
- Zyban (bupropion HCl)

In 2007, the Food and Drug Administration Amendments Act of 2007 (FDAAA) created a new section of the Food, Drug and Cosmetic Act which authorizes the FDA to require a risk evaluation and mitigation strategy (REMS) when necessary to ensure that the benefits of a drug outweigh the risks. The potential use of MedGuides as part of this mitigation strategy rapidly became popular. As of January 2011 over 150 different drug products were required to be dispensed with MedGuides as part of a REMS program.

Under the REMS program, if a drug product requires the use of a MedGuide, the patient must be provided with the MedGuide under the following circumstances:

- When the patient or the patient's agent requests a Medication Guide.
- When a drug is dispensed in an outpatient setting (e.g. a retail pharmacy or a hospital ambulatory care pharmacy) and the product will then be used by the patient without direct supervision by a health care professional.
- The first time a drug is dispensed to a health care professional for administration to a patient in an outpatient setting, such as in a clinic or dialysis or infusion center.
- The first time a drug is dispensed in an outpatient setting of any kind
- After a MedGuide is materially changed (e.g. after addition of a new indication or new safety information).
- When a drug is subject to a REMS that includes a specific requirement for reviewing or providing a MedGuide as part of an element to assure safe use.

Drug Product Substitution

The regulations that describe the process of substitution of one drug product for another are within the jurisdiction of individual states. Candidates should carefully review the mechanisms and limitations of substitution for pharmacists in the state(s) in which they are attempting to be licensed.

The premise of simple substitution is to provide a lower cost drug product in place of the drug product prescribed. A key factor in substitution has been the necessity that the originally prescribed drug and the substituted drug products had to be PHARMACEUTICALLY equivalent. That is, each drug product must have the same active ingredient, same dosage form, same route of administration, and must be identical in dosage strength or concentration. Pharmaceutically equivalent products may, however, contain different excipients.

The term, THERAPEUTIC equivalence is used to denote drug products that are

- pharmaceutical equivalents AND
- bioequivalent.

Drug products that are considered to be bioequivalent have been clinically evaluated and have been shown to have similar pharmacokinetic properties. That is, a similar ADME pathway. ADME is the acronym for

- Absorption
- Distribution
- Metabolism
- Elimination

Data submitted to the FDA by a manufacturer will include graphs that illustrate that two products containing the same drug have similar blood concentration versus time curves. Most critical in claiming bioequivalence is that two products each produce similar

- time to peak.
- peak concentrations.
- area under the curve (AUC).

The FDA will generally approve the marketing of competing drug products if they are shown not to present bioequivalence problems or, if they do present a potential problem, they are shown to meet appropriate bioequivalence standards.

A third designation, "pharmaceutical alternatives", refers to drug products that contain the same therapeutic moiety BUT may consist of different

- salts
- esters or complexes
- dosage forms
- strengths

Most states do not allow substitution among pharmaceutical alternatives, so they will not be considered in this Guide.

While simple drug substitution is self-explanatory, the term "therapeutic substitution" is more complex. This term is used when a pharmacy has the right to substitute a different drug for the one designated on the prescription or medical order, without contacting the prescriber (e.g. one cephalosporin drug for another). This practice is generally limited to institutions that utilize a drug formulary.

A committee within the institution (usually the Pharmacy and Therapeutics Committee) generally determines which drug products will be included in the formulary. All participating prescribers agree to abide by the approved therapeutic substitution policies. The intent of the drug formulary is to save the institution money by utilizing more economical drug products in a certain therapeutic area and also by reducing the need for the institution to maintain a large drug inventory.

The term "closed formulary" refers to a formulary where only the drug products listed may be used in the institution, while the term "open formulary" is used to describe a formulary that permits some unlisted drug products to be dispensed.

When the prescriber writes a prescription or the pharmacist selects a drug product for dispensing, one of the following three types of drug names may be used:

- **Generic name** - This is the single specific name assigned to a drug by the USAN. In the United States each specific drug structure is given only one generic name. For example, ampicillin denotes a chemical that has a specific chemical structure.

- **Trade name or Brand name** - This unique name is selected by a pharmaceutical company for its own brand of a generic drug. For example, one manufacturer has selected Glucophage as a trade name for its brand of metformin hydrochloride while another manufacturer has registered the trade name of Fortamet. The purpose of a brand name is to encourage prescribers to prescribe a specific company's product exclusively. Remember that every drug product that has been given a trade name or a brand name still has the same, original generic name as every other drug product containing the same active ingredient.

Some prescribers will write both the generic name and the manufacturer's name on a prescription (e.g. metformin hydrochloride - Bristol Myers Squibb). When this occurs, the pharmacist must realize that this is equivalent to writing either a trade name or brand name. In this example, the pharmacist is obligated to dispense Bristol Myers Squibb's metformin hydrochloride product.

A new drug product will often have patent protection for a number of years. Its manufacturer has exclusive rights for marketing the drug product and has likely chosen a trade name for the product. The drug product may be referred to as a "Single Source Product" since no other manufacturer markets the same drug. Once the patent has expired, other companies may submit ANDAs to gain approval for their marketing of the same drug. They may choose to use only the generic name or they may select their own exclusive brand name. When more than one manufacturer has a drug product on the market, the term "Multisource Product" is used.

Since pharmacokinetic data for new drug products are sent to the FDA for review, it is logical that the FDA will supply health professionals with bioequivalence information. A resource containing this information is known as *Approved Drug Products with Therapeutic Equivalence Evaluations*, better known as the "*The Orange Book*". This resource is published annually and updated periodically during each year. An Internet version of this resource, known as " The Electronic Orange Book" is updated continuously. There are several other reference sources available for determining the status of a specific drug product. These include:

- *United States Pharmacopeia Dispensing Information (USP/DI) Volume III* plus supplements
- *Facts and Comparisons, Inc.*
- *FDA's Internet Web site: http://www.fda.gov*

Whenever an innovator's new drug product is developed and submitted with a New Drug Application (NDA), it becomes the reference standard. Manufacturers interested in marketing a product that attempts to duplicate the innovator's drug product must submit to the FDA an Abbreviated New Drug Application (ANDA).

The bioequivalence of the generic versions of an innovator's drug product must be determined. Based upon such testing, generic products are classified in one of two categories:

- **"A" rated products** - Such products are determined to be bioequivalent to the innovator's drug product and are thus "therapeutically equivalent" to the brand name or reference product.
- **"B" rated products** - These are products that are found NOT to be bioequivalent to the innovators drug product.

Products that are A-rated may be substituted for one another while B-rated products cannot. Most states, however, limit substitution to interchanges between products that are the same dosage form. That is, one cannot substitute a capsule dosage form with a tablet dosage form or an ointment for a cream. Also, most sustained-release or controlled-release dosage forms are not interchangeable.

To further clarify the meaning of these codes, products assigned the "A" code are generally placed into one of several subcategories that generally designate different dosage forms. These subcategories include:

- **AA** - Drug products in conventional dosage forms
- **AN** - Solutions and powders for aerosolization
- **AO** - Injectable products with oil solvents
- **AP** - Injectable solutions with water as a solvent
- **AT** - Topical products (if they are the same dosage form) – e.g. fluocinolone acetonide cream products.

> **Study Tip**
>
> It is probably not necessary to memorize these subcategories.

Some drug products identified by the FDA as having actual or potential bioequivalence problems may be acceptable substitutes if the equivalency problems have been shown to be resolved by the results of in vivo and/or in vitro studies. Such drug products are given an "AB" designation, which signifies that the product meets "necessary bioequivalence requirements".

To summarize, products with similar "A" codes and having the same dosage strength may be substituted for each other while products with "B" codes cannot.

The FDA has further expanded this code system by designating some AB products as AB1, AB2, AB3, etc. These subcategories are intended to categorize drug products, which would not have been considered bioequivalent previously, into bioequivalent groups. The best examples of the use of these subcategories are the transdermal nitroglycerin patches. Originally these were classified as "B" since their release mechanisms varied from product to product. However, they are now classified as follows:

PRODUCT	CATEGORY
Nitro-Dur transdermal (Merck Sharp Dohme) (the reference standard)	AB1
Minitran Transdermal (Medicis)	AB1
Nitroglycerin Transdermal (Mylan) (the reference standard)	AB2
Nitroglycerin Transdermal (Hercon)	AB2

Thus Nitro-Dur and Minitran transdermal systems are considered bioequivalent to one another and the two generic nitroglycerin transdermal systems (Mylan and Hercon) are considered bioequivalent to one another. However, one cannot substitute an AB1 product such as Nitro-Dur or Minitran for the Mylan or Hercon generic transdermal products that are designated as AB2.

Another group of drug products with fairly lenient substitution regulations is the amino acid solutions used for preparing TPN solutions. These are classified as exceptions to the bioequivalence regulations. Such solutions may vary slightly in composition from one another, but it is unlikely that there would be significant differences in therapeutic activity between them as long as the total percentage of amino acids is the same in each. The pharmacist is permitted to substitute such amino acids solutions relatively freely.

As mentioned previously, the "B" codes are assigned to drug products that the FDA does not currently consider to be THERAPEUTICALLY equivalent to other PHARMACEUTICALLY equivalent products. Since bioequivalence problems often stem from dosage form problems, codes of BC, BD, BE, BP, BR, BS, BT, BX, and B* are sometimes assigned to such products. The meaning of these is listed below:

- **BC** - Extended-release dosage forms (capsules, tablets, injectables)
- **BD** - Active ingredients and dosage forms with documented bioequivalence problems

- **BE** - Delayed-release oral dosage forms (e.g. enteric coated tablets)
- **BN** - Aerosol nebulizer drug delivery systems
- **BP** - Active ingredients and dosage forms with potential bioequivalence problems. (e.g. injectable suspensions)
- **BR** - Suppositories or enemas that are intended for systemic absorption
- **BS** - Products that have drug standard deficiencies (e.g. a drug that contains several active components.
- **BT** - Topical products with bioequivalence issues
- **BX** - Drug products with insufficient data to determine therapeutic equivalence; also used to denote a drug product likely to lose its FDA approval

> **Study Tip**
>
> Good news! It is unlikely that any question will be asked where you must know the difference between any of the above "B" categories.

What is the status of a drug that is manufactured by the New Drug Application holder (i.e. the innovator) but is being repackaged and/or distributed by another company? Since the original company holding the NDA manufactures it, the product meets all bioequivalence requirements and will thus be considered bioequivalent.

Some drugs and their related drug products marketed before 1938 are not required to be listed in the Orange Book because they have a "Grandfather" exemption. Included in this category are drugs such as ASA with codeine, codeine, digoxin, ephedrine, epinephrine, levothyroxine, morphine, nitroglycerin, phenobarbital, oral potassium chloride preparations, pseudoephedrine, thyroid, and quinine.

In addition, some generic forms of nitroglycerin transdermal systems marketed prior to 1962 are exempt as well. While many of these products had bioavailability data, they did not have appropriate bioequivalence data. Over the past few years, however, many of these multi-source products have been listed in the Orange Book because their manufacturers recognize the value of providing substitution information.

Narrow Therapeutic Index Drugs (NTIs)

These are drugs which have narrow therapeutic ratios, i.e.

- less than a two-fold difference between the median lethal dose (LD50) and the median effective dose (ED50).
- less than a two-fold difference between the minimum toxic concentration (MTC) and the minimum effective concentration (MEC) in the blood.

Safe and effective use of such drugs requires careful titration and patient monitoring. The FDA has identified the following drugs as NTIs:

- carbamazepine
- cyclosporine
- digoxin
- ethosuximide
- levothyroxine
- lithium
- phenytoin
- procainamide
- tacrolimus
- theophylline
- warfarin.

There are ongoing studies to identify other drugs that may fall into this category.

While the FDA allows most drugs to have a variability limit of 90 to 110% of label claim, the variability limits for most NTIs are 95 to 105%. Some states have established their own tighter regulations to limit substitution of different manufacturers products.

Using the Orange Book

The Orange Book, which was originally available in book form with regular supplements, has been replaced by the Electronic Orange Book (EOB). It is available at the FDA Internet website,

http://www.fda.gov/cder/ob/default.htm

The EOB, which is continuously updated, provides interested parties with the opportunity to find and compare therapeutic equivalence (TE) codes for multi-source products.

Tables G-1-4 are abridged sections taken from the EOB. The left hand column of these tables indicates the Applicant Number. By clicking on this number, basic information about the manufacturer, approval date, and other information can be obtained. The second column from the left lists the Therapeutic Equivalence Evaluations (TE) Bioequivalence Code This is important information for the pharmacist because it indicates the bioequivalence status of each drug product. The third column from the left indicates whether or not the product is a Reference Listed Drug (RLD). RLD products are often the innovator's products that represent the standard used by new applicants to apply for an ANDA.

Tables G-1 and G-2 present abridged information about the tablet forms of the drug verapamil HCl (a generic name). Note that various dosage strengths are listed with their corresponding manufacturers. If a specific manufacturer uses a trade name or brand name, the drug product is listed by that name. Otherwise, just the generic name is listed. Note that the first oral tablet of verapamil HCl listed is Searle's Calan in 40, 80, and 120 mg strengths, all rated AB. The rest of the products listed are also rated AB. Therefore, substitution among these bioequivalent TABLET products is possible provided the same dosage strength is used.

Note that the 120 mg Calan Oral Tablet product (the only product with a "Yes" in the RLD column) was the reference standard used by the FDA for bioequivalence comparisons.

Table G-2 depicts an abridged version of the Electronic Orange

Book listing for extended-release verapamil tablet products. Note that Covera-HS is the reference standard used by the FDA for bioequivalence study comparisons. Also note that this product, manufactured by Searle, has a status of BC, indicating a lack of bioequivalence. In this case, bioequivalence problems are likely when comparing this product with the action of other extended-release verapamil products because of the special release system for the product.

TE Code	RLD	Active Ingredient	Dosage Form; Route	Strength	Proprietary Name	Applicant
AB	Yes	VERAPAMIL HCL	TABLET; ORAL	120MG	CALAN	PFIZER
AB	No	VERAPAMIL HCL	TABLET; ORAL	40MG	CALAN	PFIZER
AB	No	VERAPAMIL HCL	TABLET; ORAL	80MG	CALAN	PFIZER
AB	No	VERAPAMIL HCL	TABLET; ORAL	120MG	VERAPAMIL HCL	MYLAN
AB	No	VERAPAMIL HCL	TABLET; ORAL	80MG	VERAPAMIL HCL	MYLAN
AB	No	VERAPAMIL HCL	TABLET; ORAL	120MG	VERAPAMIL HCL	WATSON LABS
AB	No	VERAPAMIL HCL	TABLET; ORAL	40MG	VERAPAMIL HCL	WATSON LABS
AB	No	VERAPAMIL HCL	TABLET; ORAL	80MG	VERAPAMIL HCL	WATSON LABS

Table G-1 - Electronic Orange Book Listings
(abridged) for Verapamil HCl Oral Tablets

TE Code	RLD	Active Ingredient	Dosage Form; Route	Strength	Proprietary Name	Applicant
BC	Yes	VERAPAMIL HCL	TABLET; EXTENDED RELEASE; ORAL	180MG	COVERA-HS	PFIZER
BC	Yes	VERAPAMIL HCL	TABLET; EXTENDED RELEASE; ORAL	240MG	COVERA-HS	PFIZER

Table G-2 - Electronic Orange Book Listings
(abridged) for Covera-HS Tablets

Table G-3 depicts abridged Electronic Orange Book information concerning 120 mg extended-release oral capsule dosage forms of diltiazem hydrochloride. Note that some of the products on the chart are labeled AB2, AB3 or AB4. AB2 products are bioequivalent to other AB2 diltiazem hydrochloride sustained-release 120mg capsule products but are not bioequivalent with AB3 or AB4 products. Likewise, AB3 products are bioequivalent to one another but not with AB2 or AB4 products. Note that the Mylan product is associated with a BC code. It would, therefore, not be possible to substitute any other products on this chart for this one, even though this is the reference standard used by the FDA to compare these products.

What if a prescriber writes for Valeant's Cardizem CD 120 mg extended release capsule? May a pharmacist substitute with Watson's Cardia XT 120 mg product? Yes, because they are both AB3 rated AND provided that Watson's product is less expensive than Valeant's Cardizem CD product. This again relates to the fact that ALL drug products containing the exact same drug and dosage form share the same generic name. Generic substitution means that any drug product, whether it has a generic name only or has been given a trade name or brand name, may be used as a substitute, IF it is less expensive and bioequivalent.

TE Code	RLD	Active Ingredient	Dosage Form; Route	Strength	Proprietary Name	Applicant
AB2	No	DILTIAZEM HCl	CAPSULE; EXTENDED RELEASE; ORAL	120MG	DILTIAZEM HCL	APOTEX
AB3	No	DILTIAZEM HCl	CAPSULE; EXTENDED RELEASE; ORAL	120MG	CARDIA XT	WATSON
AB3	No	DILTIAZEM HCl	CAPSULE; EXTENDED RELEASE; ORAL	120MG	CARDIZEM CD	VALEANT
AB4	No	DILTIAZEM HCl	CAPSULE; EXTENDED RELEASE; ORAL	120MG	DILTZAC	APOTEX
AB4	No	DILTIAZEM HCl	CAPSULE; EXTENDED RELEASE; ORAL	120MG	DILTIAZEM HCL	SUN PHARMA
BC	Yes	DILTIAZEM HCl	CAPSULE; EXTENDED RELEASE; ORAL	120MG	DILTIAZEM HCL	MYLAN

Table G-3 - Electronic Orange Book listing (abridged) of diltiazem HCl extended release oral capsule products.

The principles explained above apply to other dosage forms as well. For example, Table G-4 depicts Electronic Orange Book listings for phenytoin oral suspension and oral chewable tablets. Note that all of the phenytoin suspension products have the same strength and have the same AB rating, with Dilantin-125 as the reference standard. Therefore, all of these products are considered to be bioequivalent to one another. There are only two oral chewable 50mg tablet products listed. The PFIZER product is the reference standard and the MYLAN product is a bioequivalent product.

TE Code	RLD	Active Ingredient	Dosage Form; Route	Strength	Proprietary Name	Applicant
AB	No	PHENYTOIN	Suspension; Oral	125MG/5ML	PHENYTOIN	TARO
AB	No	PHENYTOIN	Suspension; Oral	125MG/5ML	PHENYTOIN	WOCK-HARDT
AB	Yes	PHENYTOIN	Suspension; Oral	125MG/5ML	DILANTIN-125	PFIZER
AB	No	PHENYTOIN	Suspension; Oral	125MG/5ML	PHENYTOIN	VISTA-PHARM
AB	Yes	PHENYTOIN	Tablet, Chewable; Oral	50MG	DILANTIN	PFIZER
AB	No	PHENYTOIN	Tablet, Chewable; Oral	50MG	PHENYTOIN	MYLAN

Table G-4 - Electronic Orange Book listing (abridged) of phenytoin suspension and phenytoin chewable tablets.

Most states originally prohibited or discouraged the substitution of sustained-release, delayed-release, and other dosage forms where there may have been bioequivalence problems. However, in some cases, pharmaceutical companies have submitted data showing bioequivalence for some of these dosage forms. The pharmacist must carefully review the data presented in the Electronic Orange Book to ascertain the exact status of a drug product.

Sample Questions

1. Which of the following designations indicate that drug products of the same strength and dosage form may be interchangeable?

   I. A

   II. AB

   III. B

   (A) I only (B) III only (C) I & II only
   (D) II & III only (E) I, II, & III

2. The Electronic Orange Book uses the abbreviation RLD to indicate

   (A) a bioequivalence problem.
   (B) no bioequivalence problem.
   (C) that the drug product is used as the reference standard.
   (D) the least expensive drug product.
   (E) the drug product that is preferred by most pharmacists for substitution.

Answers: (1) C (2) C

Generic Substitution of Biosimilars

[Biologics Price Competition and Innovation Act (BPCIA) of 2009]

As part of the Patient Protection and Affordable Care Act, Congress passed the BPCIA. This act includes an approval process modeled after the process for generic small-molecule drugs under the Hatch-Waxman Act. However, the approval of new molecular biological entities are approved by one of two pathways:

351(a) pathway - A Biologic License Application (BLA) which involves a full evaluation of purity, safety, and potency.

351(k) pathway - A Biosimilar Application which invokes an abbreviated evaluation of purity, safety, and potency.

The designation of "biosimilars" refer to unique biologic drugs derived from living organisms by recombinant technology. They present new considerations for regulation. Decisions must be made concerning:

1. naming of biosimilars
2. indications for use
3. whether they may be interchangeable with similar drug products.

The FDA defines a biosimilar as a biologic product that is "highly similar" to the reference product. The reference product may be a vaccine, blood or blood component, gene therapy, tissues, or proteins (except those that are chemically synthesized polypeptides). The biosimilar product must have same mechanism of action, route of administration, dosage form and strength as the reference product. Thus no clinically meaningful difference should exist between the biosimilar and the reference product in respect to safety, purity, and potency.

To develop a biologic a manufacturer creates a unique cell line which is cloned from a single cell. Each cell line has innate properties that may lead to differences in both production and manufacturing capabilities. Among the first biologic therapy was Humulin, developed in 1982 by using recombinant DNA technology to altering E. coli through fermentation processes thus producing biosynthetic human insulin.

Mailing of Prescription Drugs

There are virtually no restrictions on mailing prescription products via the United States Postal Service (USPS). At one time controlled substances that were narcotics could not be mailed, but that regulation has been eliminated. The USPS still has regulations that prohibit mailing of poisons or alcohol-containing products that could be considered beverages.

United States Postal Services regulations permit the mailing of controlled substances by drug manufacturers or their agents, pharmacies, or other authorized handlers when distribution is lawful under DEA regulations and if the mailer or the addressee meets one of the following conditions:

- The mailer or the addressee is registered with the DEA.
- The mailer or the addressee is exempt from DEA registration as permissible by law.

United States Postal Service regulations permit mailing of any controlled substance, provided it is not outwardly dangerous and will not cause injury to a person's life or health, and if the following preparation and packaging standards are met:

- The inner container of any parcel containing controlled substances is packaged and labeled as required by the provisions of the Controlled Substances Act
- The controlled substance is placed in a plain outer container or is securely wrapped in plain paper.
- If the controlled substance consists of prescription medicines, the inner container is also labeled to show the name and address of the pharmacy, practitioner, or other person dispensing the prescription.
- The outside wrapper or container is free of markings that would indicate the nature of the contents.

USPS regulations do not apply to commercial shippers such as UPS and FedEx. These private companies may establish their own rules for mailing drug products.

Sample Questions

1. The major objective of the Electronic Orange Book is to compare drug products that are

   (A) official in the *USP/NF.*

   (B) multi-source.

   (C) chemically unique.

   (D) most economical.

   (E) therapeutically unique.

2. Colonial Labs is the first company to develop and market a particular product as a transdermal patch. This product would probably be described in the Orange Book as:

   I. NTI.

   II. A rated.

   III. the reference drug product.

   (A) I only (B) III only (C) I & II only
   (D) II & III only (E) I, II, & III

3. Certain drug products are exempt from the requirements of demonstrating therapeutic equivalence because of:

   I. the grandfather clause.

   II. their narrow therapeutic index.

   III. their high therapeutic index.

   (A) I only (B) III only (C) I & II only
   (D) II & III only (E) I, II, & III

4. Major objectives for developing a formulary include

   I. Reducing drug inventory

   II. Allowing therapeutic substitution

   III. Giving prescribers greater latitude for drug selection

   (A) I only (B) III only (C) I & II only
   (D) II & III only (E) I, II, & III

5. Therapeutic substitution is permitted only if an institution is:

   (A) nonprofit.

   (B) for profit.

   (C) using a formulary system.

   (D) under the supervision of a Pharm.D.

   (E) approved to do so by the FDA.

6. Substitution is permitted for drug products with which of the following codes?

   I. A

   II. AB

   III. B

   (A) I only (B) III only (C) I & II only

   (D) II & III only (E) I, II, & III

7. Which of the following reference sources contain(s) significant information concerning bioequivalence of drug products?

   I. *Orange Book*

   II. *USP DI*

   III. *USP/NF*

   (A) I only (B) III only (C) I & II only

   (D) II & III only (E) I, II, & III

8. Which of the following volumes of the USP DI contain(s) significant information concerning bioequivalence of drug products?

   I. Volume I

   II. Volume II

   III. Volume III

   (A) I only (B) III only (C) I & II only

   (D) II & III only (E) I, II, & III

9. A pharmacist has filled two prescriptions for controlled substances. The patient asks the pharmacist to mail the filled prescription medication to him in another state by first class mail. Which of the following is true?

(A) The pharmacist is not permitted to mail controlled substances to a patient.

(B) Only Schedule III-V medications may be mailed to a patient.

(C) Only Schedule V medications may be mailed to a patient.

(D) The outside of the package containing the controlled substances must indicate the names of the medications enclosed.

(E) None of the above choices are correct.

10. Characteristics of a drug classified as having a Narrow Therapeutic Index include which of the following?

I. Small difference between median lethal dose and median effective dose.

II. Wide variation in accuracy of chemical assays for the drug.

III. Large difference between median lethal dose and smallest therapeutically effective dose.

(A) I only (B) III only (C) I & II only
(D) II & III only (E) I, II, & III

11. All of the following drugs are classified as having Narrow Therapeutic Indexes EXCEPT:

(A) amoxicillin (B) digoxin (C) levothyroxine
(D) phenytoin (E) warfarin

Answers:

(1) B (2) B (3) A (4) C (5) C
(6) C (7) C (8) B (9) E (10) A (11) A

OBRA 90 and Patient Counseling

Portions of OBRA 90 directly impact upon pharmaceutical dispensing and care. The Medicaid Prudent Pharmaceutical Purchasing Provisions of this Act establish conditions for the federal government to reimburse states for outpatient Medicaid services. In order for a state to receive money for its Medicaid program, it must have a drug use or drug utilization review (DUR) program. The DUR program must include a prospective component (i.e. one that examines future drug use) and a retrospective program (i.e. one that examines past drug use).

> **Note**
>
> Remember that the Centers for Medicare and Medicaid Services (CMS) controls and administers Medicare while Medicaid programs are primarily administered by the individual states.

The prospective DUR is a review of a patient's written medical record and/or his medication profile before dispensing a prescription to the patient. The pharmacist must make a reasonable effort to create or update a patient medication profile each time a prescription is filled. Minimally, the following information is required in the profile:

- Patient's name, address, telephone number
- Age or date of birth
- The sex of the patient
- Disease state(s) information, if known or provided by the patient or their physician
- Any known allergies
- A list of medications previously dispensed
- Pharmacist comments concerning the patient's drug therapy,

when appropriate

Patients may refuse to divulge any or all of the above information, but the pharmacist should create or refer to the patient's medication profile and indicate the patient's refusal to provide information.

When a prescription is presented to the pharmacist, he or she must perform a prospective DUR. This consists of:

- a review of the prescription and patient records for over or under utilization of drugs.
- checking for therapeutic duplication.
- checking for incorrect doses or dosing regimens.
- extending a verbal offer to the client or to their representative to personally discuss matters that will enhance or optimize their drug therapy.

A critical portion of OBRA 90 that affects dispensing pharmacists is the requirement that an offer to counsel the patient must be provided. The OBRA 90 legislation specifically provides for patient counseling for Medicaid patients. Since Medicaid is under the jurisdiction of the individual states, each state has the right to establish whether patient counseling will be required for all patients. Most states have taken the realistic stand that all patients should be provided with the opportunity to be counseled. Most state boards of pharmacy have or are in the process of establishing standards of care, which require active verbal offers of counseling, not just a check-off system performed by a clerk.

What type of information must the pharmacist provide if counseling is requested? Federal law does not state how much or what specific information is to be provided by the pharmacist. Instead, pharmacists must use their professional judgment to determine the type and extent of information to provide. Appropriate information could include:

- The name and use of the drug
- The route of administration and duration of drug therapy

- Any special directions or cautions for taking the drug
- Common adverse effects that may be experienced
- How the patient may evaluate the effectiveness of his/her drug therapy
- How the drug should be stored and when it should be discarded
- Whether the prescription may be refilled
- What the patient should do if a dose is missed

Note

Remember. These are only examples of some of the information that the pharmacist may supply. None of these items is absolutely required and the counseling session could include anything the pharmacist considers necessary. Obviously the pharmacist should always inquire if the patient has further questions.

When does the pharmacist NOT have to counsel a patient? Only if the patient refuses to be counseled.

May a pharmacy intern counsel a patient? The utilization of pharmacy interns to counsel patients is a decision made by each state board of pharmacy. Most have included patient counseling as a function of registered pharmacy interns.

The retrospective drug utilization review is a requirement for individual states. It is not for pharmacies. It is expected that each state will establish a committee consisting of physicians, pharmacists, and other health professionals. This board or committee reviews the use of certain drugs over a period of time to ascertain whether appropriate therapy is being utilized. Obviously, the retrospective DUR is performed after prescriptions have been dispensed and information concerning the prescriptions has been sent to a clearinghouse - usually the state's Medicaid center. The DUR board may recommend that some prescribing habits of physicians be changed. The board may also initiate educational programs for both physicians and pharmacists.

OBRA 90 also established and funded demonstration projects with the intent of evaluating outcomes of patient care and the cost efficiency of pharmacist interventions.

Another objective of the OBRA 90 legislation is to reduce the cost of state Medicaid programs. Pharmaceutical manufacturers are required to offer Medicaid programs the lowest price ("best price") for drug products. If the price being charged is higher than the price charged to any other group, the company must offer a rebate of the difference to the state Medicaid program.

Health Insurance Portability & Accountability Act (HIPAA)

The basic intention of this act is to assure the security and privacy of patients' medical records while allowing the flow of health information needed to provide high quality health care. Every health care provider who **electronically** transmits health information is a covered entity. The rule is intended to limit the use, requests for, or disclosure of protected health information (PHI). Pharmacists should be aware that such privacy includes prescriptions, patient record systems (patient's prescription profiles) and recorded pharmacist comments relevant to patient therapy. While most states already have regulations concerning the confidentiality of patient medical records, the Federal Act provides for substantial fines for breaks in confidentiality. In other words, patient records must be secure and not readily available to anyone who has no reason to review them.

Medical groups such as clinics, hospitals, physician offices, etc. must provide a written privacy notice to each patient. This notice describes how medical information concerning the patient may be used and disclosed. It also advises the patient as to how he/she can get access to the information. Most groups will require the patient to sign an acknowledgment that the notice was provided. This signed form must be kept for a minimum of six years, but there is no requirement for future signatures. The organization's "HIPAA Privacy Officer" is responsible for training all medical personnel concerning the HIPAA requirements.

How does the HIPAA affect pharmacies?

HIPAA laws require that pharmacies maintain the privacy of each patient's protected health information ("PHI"). A "Notice of Privacy Practices" must be given to each patient when first provided service in the pharmacy. Ideally, the pharmacy should receive and retain an acknowledgement that the above notice was given. Other requirements include the following:

1. If the patient refuses to sign an acknowledgment, the pharmacy can still provide the service. However the pharmacist should document his/her good faith efforts to obtain an acknowledgment from the patient.
2. The acknowledgment is needed only the first time service is provided. Thus, there is no need for the patient to sign an acknowledgment every time a prescription is dispensed, and there is no expiration date for the acknowledgement. Also, only one acknowledgment is needed within a pharmacy chain.
3. A third party, such as parent or guardian, may sign the acknowledgment. Friends or relatives may not sign but may still pick up prescriptions.

The HIPAA "privacy rule" requires that a patient consent to the sharing of private data. Obviously blanket "consent" forms are used by institutions, etc. to safeguard their rights to information. Also, most insurance companies require that clients sign a waiver allowing the company to process and audit medical and prescription claims. When information concerning several patients is being accumulated, a "de-identification" process must be considered. For example, when publishing a research paper or giving a seminar presentation, individual patient names, addresses or other identifications must be removed.

Patients may report perceived violations of the HIPAA to the Department of Health and Human Services Office for Civil Rights (HHS/OCR). Also, law suits known as "qui tam" lawsuits may be brought by whistle-blowers under the False Claims Act by private citizens who are aware of fraud against the federal government. Whistleblowers that are employees or business associates of entities covered by HIPAA, may disclose PHI if, in good faith, they believe unlawful or potentially dangerous practices toward patients are being conducted. If such individuals divulge knowledge to boards of pharmacy or to the DHHS, their employers cannot retaliate against them.

Since pharmacies must also adhere to the HIPAA requirements, patients should be notified about their privacy rights and how their health care information (medical histories and prescriptions records) may be used. The pharmacy must post its entire "Notice of Privacy Practices" in a prominent location and on its web site if one exists. When a service is first initiated with a new patient, the patient must be informed of the privacy provisions used by the pharmacy. Ideally a written acknowledgment, from the patient, of receipt of the notice should be obtained, but having the patient sign or initial the prescription log book is acceptable provided the patient is informed of the purpose of the signature. All family members do not have to receive the notice; instead just the person named in an insurance policy. Thus, children under the age of 18 do not have to sign the privacy notice. A record of required signatures must be maintained for six years from date obtained or from the last date a prescription is dispensed (whichever is later).

Patient records must be held secure. Theoretically, the only parties that should have access to a specific prescription or patient prescription records are the individual patient, the pharmacist and auxiliary personnel authorized to fill or read a prescription, the prescriber and his/her personnel, and authorized legal personnel such as board of pharmacy or DEA inspectors. While it is obvious that a pharmacist should not allow pharmaceutical sales representatives or other individuals to randomly review the pharmacy's prescription files or a medication profile, other situations are more complex. For example, can the spouse of a patient see the medication profile or receive a copy of the prescription? Theoretically, the actual patient must grant written permission first. If a pharmacy mails a friendly reminder to a patient concerning the need for a refill of a prescription, it should be done in a manner in which others will not see the drug name or therapeutic use. The name of a drug or its use should not be provided upon telephone request unless the pharmacist is certain that the patient has agreed to the request.

Consultations with the patient concerning prescriptions must be conducted in a manner that minimizes chance of incidental disclosures to other persons who may be nearby. Communications over the telephone should be conducted so that unauthorized persons will not overhear conversations. It is permissible to leave messages on answering machines or with a family member provided only "minimally necessary" information is provided. It is also permissible for the pharmacist using his/her professional judgment to allow a relative or friend to pick up a filled prescription. It is not necessary for the patient to give written permission or to provide the name of the person picking up the prescription in advance.

International Commerce Involving Drugs and Drug Products

Laws and regulations for the transportation of drugs and drug products between the United States and foreign countries are both confusing and subject to change by the Congress, the FDA, or the President. Three terms that are often employed, but with somewhat ambiguous definitions, are exportation, importation, and reimportation of drug products. This book will use the following definitions:

Exportation is the shipment of drug products to a foreign country. This action is generally acceptable if performed by the original manufacturer or a duly licensed wholesaler, and if there is no intention to bring the product back into the United States.

Importation implies that a drug product is being brought into the United States from another country for distribution. Theoretically the drug product must meet all of the standards established by the FDA for that drug including the FDA's GMP and labeling standards.

Reimportation refers to a drug product that is manufactured in the United States with FDA-approved labeling, shipped to a foreign country, and then shipped back into the United States. According to the FDA, this procedure is legal only if performed by the original manufacturer.

Counterfeit Drugs

Because of the possibility that counterfeit prescription drugs may be available in foreign countries, the FDA and other agencies oppose the purchase of prescription drugs from abroad. They also warn against purchase of such drug products from domestic web sites unless they display the VIPPS (Verified Internet Pharmacy Practice Sites) seal. Developed by the National Association of Boards of Pharmacy (NABP), this hyperlink seal, when clicked by a consumer, allows the visitor to link to the NABP VIPPS site where verified information about the pharmacy is available.

Out-of-state and Foreign Prescriptions

Controversial issues relate to the legality of pharmacists filling prescriptions written by prescribers in other states and in foreign countries and Americans who obtain prescription drugs from other countries.

The legality of filling of prescriptions written by prescribers in other states or foreign countries is not a clear issue. Most individual states have regulations, which define which health professionals may diagnose, treat, dispense, and prescribe. Often the regulations specify that only licensed practitioners may write prescriptions, with the understanding that pharmacies will fill only those prescriptions written within the state. However, current practice often entails filling out-of-state prescriptions. The prime consideration for the pharmacist is to establish that the prescriber, the patient and the prescription are legitimate. Using his/her professional judgment, the pharmacist should ascertain the legitimacy of each prescription received.

As a rule, the FDA prohibits the interstate shipment (which includes importation) of unapproved new drugs. Unapproved new drugs are any drugs, including foreign-made versions of U.S. approved drugs, that have not received FDA approval to demonstrate they meet the federal requirements for safety and effectiveness. It is the importer's obligation to demonstrate to FDA that any drugs offered for importation have been approved by FDA.

A side issue relates to whether a pharmacy may fill a foreign prescription and directly export it to a foreign country. This appears to be legitimate if the prescription is for a reasonable quantity of drug. It should be remembered that prescription drugs must be used under the supervision of a prescriber. In filling foreign prescriptions or mailing drug products to other countries it becomes difficult for the pharmacist to determine whether or not a patient is being properly monitored.

Note

NONE of the above statements apply to controlled substances. Federal regulations require that only practitioners licensed to practice in the United States may write prescriptions for controlled substances.

Another current issue relates to the issue of some individuals who obtain prescription drugs from outside the United States via the mail or by visiting another country. The FDA does not sanction such actions but appears to be somewhat flexible provided that

1. The intended use of the drug is unapproved and is for a serious condition for which effective treatment may not be available domestically either through commercial or clinical means;
2. The drug product will not be distributed to others;
3. The product is considered not to represent an unreasonable risk;
4. The individual seeking to import the product affirms in writing that it is for the patient's own use (generally not more than a 3 month supply) and provides the name and address of the doctor licensed in the U.S. responsible for his or her treatment with the product, or provides evidence that the product is for the continuation of a treatment begun in a foreign country/area.
5. The drug supply may be shipped directly to the patient or to either their physician or pharmacy.

It should be remembered that even if all of these factors are present, the drugs still remain illegal and the FDA may decide that such drugs should be refused entry or seized.

In addition, the FDA has stated that businesses such as Internet pharmacies must sell only FDA-approved drugs, including those manufactured in foreign countries. This means that the drug product must meet ALL FDA standards for manufacturing, ingredients, formulations, etc.

Elcctronic Prescribing

Electronic prescribing is a way for prescribers to send prescriptions electronically and directly to a pharmacy. It is becoming increasingly popular because it can save expense, time, and medication errors.

Prescribers will also have secure access to a patience medication history as well as potential drug interactions, allergies, and other warnings.

States such as New York have already instituted a universal requirement for electronic prescriptions. There is little doubt that other states will move in the same direction.

Sample Questions

1. What constitutes appropriate action for a pharmacist when an uncooperative patient refuses to provide information for his patient prescription profile?

   I. The pharmacist should explain that it is illegal for the patient to refuse to provide the requested information.

   II. The pharmacist may fill the prescription without a medication history.

   III. The pharmacist may refuse to fill the prescription.

   (A) I only (B) III only (C) I & II only
   (D) II & III only (E) I, II, & III

2. Which of the following might represent a breach of privacy based upon the federal Health Insurance Portability and Accountability Act (HIPAA)?

   I. Allowing a pharmaceutical sales representative to examine your prescription files to ascertain if a certain doctor is prescribing their company's new antidepressant.

   II. Sending a postcard reminding a patient that his Prozac prescription needs to be refilled.

   III. Providing a husband with a list of drug products and their therapeutic uses, received by his wife last year.

   (A) I only (B) III only (C) I & II only
   (D) II & III only (E) I, II, & III

3. According to FDA guidelines, which of the following activities are NOT acceptable for an individual receiving mailed prescription drug products from a Canadian pharmacy?

   I. Having the drug mailed directly to his home rather than to his physician.

   II. Receiving a six months supply of the drug product.

   III. Splitting the drug supply with his neighbor, who has a prescription for the same product.

   (A) I only (B) III only (C) I & II only
   (D) II & III only (E) I, II, & III

4. A police officer visits a pharmacy and informs the pharmacist that he has arrested an individual suspected of writing a fictitious prescription that was filled in the pharmacy. The officer requests the original prescription as evidence. Which of the following would be appropriate action(s) for the pharmacist to take?

   I. The pharmacist should give the officer the prescription as long as the officer provides the pharmacist with a written receipt.

   II. As described, the prescription is not legally considered to be a forged prescription.

   III. The pharmacist is not obligated to give the officer the prescription.

   (A) I only (B) III only (C) I & II only
   (D) II & III only (E) I, II, & III

5. Under the Poison Prevention Packaging Act (PPPA), the use of closures that are "reversible", i.e. not child-resistant in one direction but child-resistant in the opposite position is

(A) permitted only for use in prescriptions intended for geriatric patients.
(B) illegal.
(C) discouraged but not prohibited under the PPPA.
(D) permitted only for use in nursing homes.
(E) permitted only for use in hospice patients.

6. A client presents a prescription for an antidiabetic drug written for his cousin living in France. Which one of the following actions is MOST appropriate for the pharmacist to take?

(A) Refuse to fill the prescription stating that the condition is not life-threatening.
(B) Fill the prescription after obtaining a written guarantee that the drug will be shipped abroad.
(C) Fill the prescription using professional judgment to determine that it is a legitimate prescription.
(D) Refuse to fill the prescription stating that both federal and state laws prohibits such dispensing.
(E) Fill the prescription after obtaining permission from the FDA.

7. How often must a pharmacy have a patient sign a new notice that he/she has been informed of the pharmacy's privacy practices?

(A) Every time a new prescription is filled.

(B) Every time a refill is dispensed.

(C) Every 6 months.

(D) Every year.

(E) There is no such requirements in HIPAA regulations.

8. A customer had a prescription originally filled on December 1, 2015 and acknowledged receiving the pharmacy's notice of privacy rights under HIPAA. She also receives a refill dispensed on January 2, 2016. What is the earliest date that the pharmacy may discard the patient's acknowledgment?

(A) 12/1/2016 (B) 1/2/2017 (C) 12/1/2021

(D) 1/2/2022 (E) never

9. A pharmaceutical manufacturer requests from a community pharmacy the names and addresses of patients receiving the company's antidepressant product so that special discount coupons may be provided to the patients. This scenario is probably in violation of which of the following laws?

(A) DSHEA

(B) FDA Modernization Act of 1997

(C) HIPAA

(D) OBRA

(E) Sherman Antitrust Act

10. A pharmacist telephones a patient's home to advise him of the upcoming need to refill one of his prescriptions. With which of the following parties may the message be left?

I. patient's wife

II. patient's mother

III. patient's brother-in-law

(A) I only (B) III only (C) I & II only

(D) II & III only (E) I, II, & III

11. A pharmacy practitioner is preparing a research paper dealing with the side effects of LMW heparins in 20 of her patients. Which of the following patient information must be removed from the paper before submission for publication?

I. home address

II. social security number

III. age

(A) I only (B) III only (C) I & II only

(D) II & III only (E) I, II, & III

12. The term used in the HIPAA Privacy Rules to describe the above action is:

(A) debriefing

(B) depersonalization

(C) document erasure

(D) de-indentification

(E) anti-terrorist protection

13. A pharmacy student's aunt asks for a good online pharmacy site so she can reduce the cost of her prescription drugs. Which one of the following sources may provide the most reliable information?

(A) APhA (B) ASHP (C) Chamber of Commerce

(D) VIPPS (E) USP DI

14. The Biologic Price Competition and Innovation Act is utilized to market which of the following types of drugs?

I. biosimilars

II. vaccines

III. orphan drugs

(A) I only (B) III only (C) I & II only

(D) II & III only (E) I, II, & III

15. Two drug products may be considered biosimilar even if they differ in which one of the following characteristics?

(A) molecular structure (B) potency (C) purity

(D) therapeutic use (E) route of administration

Answers:

(1) D (2) E (3) D (4) D (5) C (6) C

(7) E (8) D (9) C (10) E (11) C

(12) D (13) D (14) C (15) A

Section H

Controlled Substances

Definitions Related to Controlled Substances

The following definitions are listed in the Controlled Substances Act (CSA). While candidates are not required to write out definitions on the MPJE®, they are expected to be able to understand these terms when they are used in questions. Of particular importance are definitions that include lists of drugs. Candidates should review these lists carefully and be able to identify drugs listed in questions. Candidates should not try to memorize any of these definitions, but review them so they are somewhat familiar.

ACT - The Controlled Substances Act and/or the Controlled Substances Import and Export Act as amended periodically.

ADDICT - Any individual who habitually uses any narcotic drug so as to endanger the public morals, health, safety, or welfare, or who is so far addicted to the use of narcotic drugs as to have lost the power of self-control with reference to his addiction.

> **Note**
>
> A person who becomes habituated while using a prescribed narcotic is not generally considered to be an addict.

ADMINISTER - Refers to the direct application of a controlled substance to the body of a patient or research subject by -

(A) a practitioner (or, in his presence, by his authorized agent), or

(B) the patient or research subject at the direction and in the presence of the practitioner, whether such application be by injection, inhalation, ingestion, or any other means.

ADMINISTRATION - The Drug Enforcement Administration.

ADMINISTRATOR - The Administrator of the Drug Enforcement Administration (DEA). The Administrator has been delegated authority under the Act by the Attorney General of the United States. The Attorney General determines the schedule classification for new controlled substances.

> ***Note***
>
> Remember that DEA is under the supervision of the Attorney General of the United States.

ANABOLIC STEROID - any drug or hormonal substance, chemically and pharmacologically related to testosterone (other than estrogens, progestins, and corticosteroids) that promotes muscle growth, and includes:

- Boldenone
- Chlorotestosterone
- Dihydrotestosterone
- Drostanolone
- Ethylestrenol
- Fluoxymesterone
- Formebulone
- Mesterolone
- Methandienone
- Methandranone
- Methandriol
- Methandrostenolone
- Methenolone
- Methyltestosterone
- Mibolerone
- Nandrolone
- Norethandrolone
- Oxandrolone
- Oxymesterone
- Oxymetholone
- Stanolone
- Stanozolol
- Testolactone
- Testosterone
- Trenbolone

- Any salt, ester, or isomer of a drug or substance described or listed above, if that salt, ester, or isomer promotes muscle growth. Except such terms do not include an anabolic steroid which is expressly intended for administration through implants to cattle or other non-human species and which has been approved by the Secretary of Health and Human Services for such administration. If any person prescribes, dispenses, or distributes such steroid for human use, such person shall be considered to have prescribed, dispensed, or distributed an anabolic steroid within the meaning of this paragraph.

Study Tip

Most drugs that have anabolic steroid activity have the suffix "androlone" in them. Look for that suffix in questions related to these drugs.

COMMERCIAL CONTAINER - Any bottle, jar, tube, ampule, or other receptacle in which a substance is held for distribution or dispensing to an ultimate user. The term commercial container does not include any package liner, package insert or other material kept with or within a commercial container, nor any carton, crate, drum, or other package in which commercial containers are stored or are used for shipment of controlled substances.

COMPOUNDER - Any person engaging in maintenance or detoxification treatment who also mixes, prepares, packages or changes the dosage form of a narcotic drug listed in Schedules II, III, IV or V for use in maintenance or detoxification treatment by another narcotic treatment program.

CONTROLLED SUBSTANCE - A drug or other substance, or immediate precursor, included in schedule I, II, III, IV, or V of the CSA. The term does not include distilled spirits, wine, malt beverages, or tobacco.

DETOXIFICATION TREATMENT - The dispensing, for a period of time as specified below, of a narcotic drug or narcotic drugs in decreasing doses to an individual to alleviate adverse physiological or psychological effects as part of their withdrawal from the continuous or sustained use of a narcotic drug. Such programs are intended to bring the individual to a narcotic drug-free state within such period of time. There are two types of detoxification treatment - short-term and long-term.

- Short-term detoxification treatment is for a period not in excess of 30 days.
- Long-term detoxification treatment is for a period greater than 30 days but not in excess of 180 days.

DISPENSE - To deliver a controlled substance to an ultimate user or research subject by, or pursuant to the lawful order of, a practitioner, including the prescribing and administering of a controlled substance and the packaging, labeling or compounding necessary to prepare the substance for such delivery.

DISPENSER - A practitioner who delivers a controlled substance to an ultimate user or research subject.

DRUG - (A) Articles recognized in the *United States Pharmacopoeia/National Formulary* (*USP/NF*), *Homeopathic Pharmacopoeia of the United States* (*HPUS*), or any supplement to them; and (B) Articles intended for use in the diagnosis, cure, mitigation, treatment, or prevention of disease in man or other animals; and (C) Articles (other than food) intended to affect the structure or any function of the body of humans or other animals.

EXPORT - Taking out or removal of drugs listed in the CSA from the jurisdiction of the United States.

EXPORTER - includes every person who exports, or who acts as an export broker for exportation of controlled substances listed in any schedule.

HEARING - (A) Any hearing held for the granting, denial, revocation, or suspension of a registration; or (B) Any hearing held to set quotas for the amount of controlled substance that may be purchased or manufactured; or (C) Any hearing held for the issuance, amendment, or repeal of any rule issued as part of the Controlled Substances Act.

IMPORT - Bringing in or introduction of a controlled substance into either the jurisdiction of the United States or the customs territory of the United States.

IMPORTER - includes every person who imports, or who acts as an import broker for importation of controlled substances listed in any schedule.

INDIVIDUAL PRACTITIONER - A physician, dentist, veterinarian, or other individual licensed, registered, or otherwise permitted, by the United States or the jurisdiction in which he/she practices, to dispense a controlled substance in the course of professional practice. This term does not include a pharmacist, a pharmacy, or an institutional practitioner.

INSTITUTIONAL PRACTITIONER - A hospital or other entity (other than an individual) licensed, registered, or otherwise permitted, by the United States or the jurisdiction in which it practices, to dispense a controlled substance in the course of professional practice. This term does not include a pharmacy.

INVENTORY - All stocks of Schedule I or II controlled substances manufactured or otherwise acquired by a registrant, whether in bulk, commercial containers, or contained in pharmaceutical preparations, and that are in the possession of the registrant.

JURISDICTION OF THE UNITED STATES - The customs territory of the United States, the Virgin Islands, the Canal Zone, Guam, American Samoa, and the Trust Territories of the Pacific Islands.

LABEL - Any display of written, printed, or graphic matter placed upon the commercial container of any controlled substance by its manufacturer.

LABELING - All labels and other written, printed, or graphic matter on any controlled substance or any of its commercial containers or wrappers. This also includes such material that accompanies such a controlled substance.

LISTED CHEMICAL - Any List I chemical or List II chemical. (See below for further clarification.)

LIST I CHEMICAL - A chemical specifically identified in the CSA that, in addition to legitimate uses, is used in manufacturing a controlled substance in violation of the CSA and is important to the manufacture of a controlled substance (e.g. pseudoephedrine, phenylpropanolamine, ergotamine, etc.).

LIST II CHEMICAL - A chemical, other than a List I chemical that, in addition to legitimate uses, is used in manufacturing a controlled substance in violation of the Act (e.g. acetone, ethyl ether, potassium permanganate).

LONG TERM CARE FACILITY (LTCF) - A nursing home, retirement care, mental care or other facility or institution which provides extended health care to resident patients.

MAINTENANCE TREATMENT - The dispensing, for a period in excess of 21 days, of a narcotic drug or narcotic drugs in the treatment of an individual for dependence upon heroin or other morphine-like drug.

MANUFACTURE

- The producing, preparation, propagation, compounding, manufacturing, or processing of a drug or other substance.
- The packaging or repackaging of such substance.
- The labeling or relabeling of the commercial container of such substance.

This definition does not include the activities of a practitioner who dispenses, prepares, compounds, packages or labels such substance in the course of his/her professional practice.

> ### Note
>
> A pharmacist that compounds a prescription as part of their professional practice is NOT considered to be manufacturing.

MID-LEVEL PRACTITIONER - An individual practitioner, OTHER than a physician, dentist, veterinarian, or podiatrist, who is licensed, registered, or otherwise permitted by the United States or the jurisdiction in which he/she practices, to dispense a controlled substance in the course of professional practice.

> ### Note
>
> Examples of mid-level practitioners include, but are not limited to, health care providers such as nurse practitioners, nurse midwives, nurse anesthetists, clinical nurse specialists and physician assistants who are authorized to dispense controlled substances by the state in which they practice.

NAME - The official, brand, common, chemical or usual name of a substance.

NARCOTIC DRUG - Any of the following drugs, no matter how they are derived or synthesized:

- Opium, opiates, derivatives of opium and opiates, including their isomers, esters, ethers, salts, and salts of isomers, esters, and ethers. Such term does not include the isoquinoline alkaloids of opium.
- Poppy straw and concentrate of poppy straw.

- Coca leaves, ***except*** coca leaves and extracts of coca leaves from which cocaine, ecgonine and derivatives of ecgonine or their salts have been removed.
- Cocaine, its salts, optical and geometric isomers, and salts of isomers.
- Ecgonine, its derivatives, their salts, isomers and salts of isomers.
- Any compound, mixture, or preparation, which contains any quantity of any of the substances referred to in this section.

NARCOTIC TREATMENT PROGRAM - A program engaged in maintenance and/or detoxification treatment with narcotic drugs.

NET DISPOSAL - For a stated period, the quantity of a Schedule I or II controlled substance distributed by the registrant to another person, plus the quantity of that substance used by the registrant in the production of (or converted by the registrant into) another Schedule I or II controlled or noncontrolled substance, plus the quantity of such drugs that are disposed of by the registrant. This quantity is reduced by any Schedule I or II drugs returned to the registrant by any purchaser, and distributed by the registrant to another registered manufacturer.

PERSON - Any individual, corporation, government or governmental subdivision or agency, business trust, partnership, association, or other legal entity.

PHARMACIST - Any pharmacist licensed by a state to dispense controlled substances, and any other person (e.g., a pharmacy intern) authorized by a state to dispense controlled substances under the supervision of a pharmacist licensed by such state.

PRESCRIPTION - An order for medication, which is dispensed to an ultimate user. This definition does not include an order for medication dispensed for immediate administration to a patient. (e.g., an order to dispense a drug for immediate administration to an inpatient in a hospital is not a prescription.)

PURCHASER - Any registered person entitled to obtain and execute order forms pursuant to the CSA.

READILY RETRIEVABLE - Records that are kept in such a manner that they can be separated out from all other records in a reasonable time.

REGISTER (REGISTRATION) - Refers only to registration required and permitted by the Controlled Substances Act.

REGISTRANT - Any person who is registered under the Controlled Substance Act.

REVERSE DISTRIBUTOR - a registrant who receives controlled substances acquired from another DEA registrant for the purpose of—

(1) Returning unwanted, unusable, or outdated controlled substances to the manufacturer or the manufacturer's agent; or

(2) Where necessary, processing such substances or arranging for processing such substances for disposal.

SCHEDULED LISTED CHEMICAL PRODUCT -

(1) A product that contains ephedrine, pseudoephedrine, or phenylpropanolamine or their salts or optical isomers, and may be marketed or distributed lawfully in the United States under the FD&C Act as a nonprescription drug.

(2) Scheduled listed chemical product does not include any product that is a controlled substance as defined in the CSA. In the absence of such scheduling by the Attorney General, a chemical specified in paragraph (1) of this definition may not be considered to be a controlled substance.

SUPPLIER - Any registered person entitled to fill order forms under the Controlled Substances Act.

VALID PRESCRIPTION - A prescription that is issued for a legitimate medical purpose by an individual practitioner licensed by law to administer and prescribe the drugs concerned and acting in the usual course of the practitioner's professional practice.

Registration of Manufacturers, Distributors, and Dispensers

Individuals (e.g. researchers), manufacturers, distributors, laboratories, exporters, narcotic treatment programs, or dispensing locations (e.g. pharmacies), which are authorized to possess controlled substances, must be registered by the DEA to engage in these activities. Hospital registrations are issued to the entire hospital as an "institutional practitioner".

> **Note**
>
> Pharmacists do not generally need to register with the DEA if they are working in a registered establishment.

At the time a retail pharmacy, hospital/clinic, practitioner or teaching institution is first registered, that business activity shall be assigned to a specific month of the year. The expiration date of the registrant will be the last day of the month designated. After the initial registration period, the registration expires 36 months from the initial expiration date.

Applications for Registration

Specific DEA registration forms must be used by different types of entities to register with the DEA. For example:

- Pharmacies – Form 224
- Manufacturers, Distributors, Importers, Exporters, or Researchers – Form 225

- Narcotic Treatment Programs - Form 363

Registration renewal forms for these entities generally have the same number, but with an "a" suffix, i.e. 224a, 225a, and 363a. These forms are mailed to each registered entity approximately 60 days before the expiration date of the registration.

If a registered entity does not receive registration renewal forms within 45 days before the expiration date of his/her registration, he/she must promptly notify DEA and request such forms in writing.

> **Note**
>
> Remember these important time periods:
>
> — A DEA registration is valid for 36 months.
>
> — Registration renewal forms are sent to the registrant 60 days before the expiration date of the registration.
>
> — Registrants must notify DEA in writing if they have not received their renewal forms within 45 days of their expiration date.

Each application must include all information called for in the form, unless the item is not applicable, in which case this fact shall be indicated.

Each application, attachment, or other document filed as part of an application, must be signed by the

- applicant, if an individual, or
- by a partner of the applicant, if a partnership, or
- by an officer of the applicant, if a corporation, corporate division, association, trust or other entity.

Note

Federal law does not require the applicant for DEA registration to be a pharmacist.

An applicant may authorize one or more individuals, who would not otherwise be authorized to do so, to sign applications for the applicant by filing with the Registration Unit of the DEA a Power of Attorney for each such individual. A person who is authorized to sign registration applications must sign the Power of Attorney. It must also contain the signature of the individual being authorized to sign applications. The Power of Attorney is valid until revoked by the applicant.

Note

Every location where controlled substances are manufactured, distributed or dispensed must have its own DEA registration EXCEPT for the following:

- Warehouses used by registrants to store controlled substances.
- A practitioner's office where drugs are prescribed, but not administered or dispensed.
- Common carriers (e.g. freight delivery companies).
- An office where sales of controlled substances are solicited, made or supervised, but the location does not contain controlled substances.

The DEA may deny registration if the Applicant has

- materially falsified the information on the application.

- been convicted of a drug-related felony.
- committed acts which would make registration inconsistent with the public interest.
- had its state license suspended, revoked or denied.

In addition, the DEA may revoke a registration for the above reasons as well as in cases where the applicant has been subject to mandatory exclusion from participation in the Medicare or state health care program.

Re-registration

Any person who is registered may apply to be re-registered not more than 60 days before the expiration date of their registration. Bulk manufacturers of Schedule I or II controlled substances or importers of Schedule I or II controlled substances may apply to be re-registered not more than 120 days before the expiration date of their registration.

Commercial Containers

Each commercial container containing a controlled substance must have printed on the label the symbol designating the product's assigned controlled substance schedule (i.e. C-II, C-III, etc.). The word "Schedule" need not be used. The symbol must be large enough to be easily seen without taking the container off the shelf.

Schedule I Controlled Substances

Drugs classified as Schedule I controlled substances are those that have the following characteristics:

- Have a high potential for abuse.
- Have no currently accepted medical use in treatment in the United States.
- Lack accepted information on the safety of their use, even un-

der medical supervision.

The following are common examples of Schedule I drugs:

- Bufotenine
- Diethylamide
- Heroin
- Lysergic acid (LSD)
- Marijuana (cannibis)
- Mescaline
- Methaqualone
- Peyote

Note

Keep your eyes on marijuana! There is a good possibility that the DEA will reschedule marijuana from Schedule I to Schedule II, thereby essentially legalizing medicinal cannabis in all 50 states with a doctors prescription.

Study Tip

Do not attempt to memorize the exhaustive list of the hundreds of compounds that DEA classifies in Schedule I. The drugs given as examples above are the drugs that you will most likely be questioned about.

Schedule II Controlled Substances

Drugs classified as Schedule II controlled substances are those that have the following characteristics:

- Have a high potential for abuse.
- Have currently accepted medical use in treatment in the United States or a currently accepted medical use with severe restrictions.
- Abuse of the drug may lead to severe physical or psychological dependence.

The following are examples of Schedule II drugs:

- Straight opiates and opioids
  - — Alfentanil (Alfenta)
  - — Cocaine
  - — Codeine
  - — Diphenoxylate
  - — Fentanyl (Sublimaze, Duragesic)
  - — Hydrocodone and hydrocodone combination products (Vicodin, Lorcet, Lortab, etc.)
  - — Hydromorphone (Dilaudid)
  - — Levomethadyl Acetate
  - — Levorphanol
  - — Meperidine (Demerol)
  - — Methadone
  - — Morphine (MS Contin, etc.)
  - — Nabilone (Cesamet)
  - — Oxycodone (OxyContin, Percodan, Percocet)
  - — Sufentanyl (Sufenta)
  - — Tincture of Opium
- Stimulants
  - — Amphetamine (Adderall, Vyvanse)
  - — Methylphenidate (Ritalin, Concerta, etc.)
  - — Methamphetamine (Desoxyn)

- Depressants
  - Pentobarbital
  - Secobarbital (Seconal)
- Hallucinogens
  - Phencyclidine (PCP)

> **Study Tip**
>
> Carefully review the drugs in Schedule II. While some are quite obscure, many are commonly used and are often a source of questions on licensing exams. Remember that Schedule II includes drugs that are straight opiates and opioids (e.g. codeine, morphine, meperidine, hydrocodone combination products (e.g. Vicodin, Lortab, etc.)) as well as amphetamine and amphetamine-like drugs, and some barbiturates.

Schedule III Controlled Substances

Drugs classified as Schedule III controlled substances are those that have the following characteristics:

- Have a potential for abuse less than that of the drugs or other substances in schedules I and II.
- Have a currently accepted medical use in treatment in the United States
- Abuse of the drug or other substance may lead to moderate or low physical dependence or high psychological dependence

The following are examples of Schedule III drugs:

- Acetaminophen w/Codeine
- Anabolic Steroids

Note

Anabolic steroids are classified in Schedule III by the federal government. Some states may classify them or other Schedule III substances in Schedule II.

Study Tip

Remember that hydrocodone products that are combinations with acetaminophen (e.g. Vicodin, Lortab, etc.), aspirin (e.g. Lortab ASA), chlorpheniramine (e.g. Tussionex), or any other combinations have been reclassified to Schedule II to reduce the abuse of such products.

- Benzphetamine (Didrex)
- Buprenorphine (Buprenex)
- Buprenorphine/Naloxone (Suboxone)
- Butabarbital (Butisol)
- Butalbital (Fiorinal) (NOT Fioricet)
- Dronabinol (Marinol)
- Nalorphine
- Phendimetrazine (Bontril)
- Any compound, mixture or preparation containing amobarbital, secobarbital, pentobarbital or their salts combined with one or more other active medicinal ingredients that are not listed in any schedule
- Any suppository dosage form containing amobarbital, secobarbital or pentobarbital or their salts.

Note

Notice that Schedule II barbiturates such as amobarbital, secobarbital, and pentobarbital become Schedule III substances if they are combined with noncontrolled drugs (e.g. aspirin) or if they are in a suppository dosage form.

- Gamma hydroxybutyrate (GHB, sodium oxybate, Xyrem)
- Narcotic Drugs. Unless specifically excepted or unless listed in another schedule, any material, compound, mixture, or preparation containing any of the following narcotic drugs, or their salts calculated as the free anhydrous base or alkaloid, in limited quantities as set forth below:

  (1) Not more than 1.8 grams of codeine per 100 milliliters or not more than 90 milligrams per dosage unit, with an equal or greater quantity of an isoquinoline alkaloid of opium.

  (2) Not more than 1.8 grams of codeine per 100 milliliters or not more than 90 milligrams per dosage unit, with one or more active, non-narcotic ingredients in recognized therapeutic amounts (e.g.Tylenol w/codeine, Empirin w/ Codeine, etc.).

  (3) Not more than 300 milligrams of dihydrocodeinone (hydrocodone) per 100 milliliters or not more than 15 milligrams per dosage unit, with a four-fold or greater quantity of an isoquinoline alkaloid of opium (e.g. Tussionex, Lortab, Vicodin).

  (4) Not more than 300 milligrams of dihydrocodeinone (hydrocodone) per 100 milliliters or not more than 15 milligrams per dosage unit, with one or more active non-narcotic ingredients in recognized therapeutic amounts.

  (5) Not more than 1.8 grams of dihydrocodeine per 100 milliliters or not more than 90 milligrams per dosage unit, with

one or more active non-narcotic ingredients in recognized therapeutic amounts (e.g. Synalgos-DC).

(6) Not more than 300 milligrams of ethylmorphine per 100 milliliters or not more than 15 milligrams per dosage unit, with one or more active, non-narcotic ingredients in recognized therapeutic amounts.

(7) Not more than 500 milligrams of opium per 100 milliliters or per 100 grams or not more than 25 milligrams per dosage unit, with one or more active, non-narcotic ingredients in recognized therapeutic amounts.

(8) Not more than 50 milligrams of morphine per 100 milliliters or per 100 grams, with one or more active, non-narcotic ingredients in recognized therapeutic amounts.

Study Tip

Note that with the exception of opium and morphine, quantities of drugs listed in the above section as Schedule III substances are all evenly divisible by THREE. This may be helpful if you are asked to determine the schedule of a compounded product.

Schedule IV Controlled Substances

Drugs classified as schedule IV controlled substances are those that have the following characteristics:

- Have a low potential for abuse relative to the drugs or other substances in schedule III.
- Have a currently accepted medical use in treatment in the United States.
- Abuse may lead to limited physical or psychological dependence relative to the drugs or other substances in Schedule III.

The following are examples of Schedule IV drugs:

- Alprazolam (Xanax)
- Butorphanol (Stadol)
- Carisoprodol (Soma)
- Chloral Hydrate
- Chlordiazepoxide (Librium)
- Clonazepam (Klonopin)
- Diazepam (Valium)
- Diethylpropion (Tenuate)
- Eszopiclone (Lunesta)
- Fenfluramine
- Flurazepam
- Mazindol
- Meprobamate
- Midazolam
- Modafinil
- Oxazepam
- Pemoline
- Pentazocine (Talwin)
- Phenobarbital
- Phentermine
- Propoxyphene
- Sibutramine
- Temazepam (Restoril)
- Tramadol (Ultram)
- Triazolam (Halcion)
- Zaleplon (Sonata)
- Zolpidem (Ambien)

Study Tip

Note that many of the drugs in the list above are benzodiazepines and end in the suffixes "azolam" or "azepam". Also, important drugs such as phenobarbital, eszopiclone, zaleplon and zolpidem are in this category.

Schedule V Controlled Substances

Drugs classified as schedule V controlled substances are those that have the following characteristics:

- Have a low potential for abuse relative to the drugs or other substances in schedule IV.
- Have a currently accepted medical use in treatment in the United States.
- Abuse of the drug or other substance may lead to limited physical or psychological dependence relative to the drugs or other substances in schedule IV.

The following are examples of Schedule V drugs:

- Narcotic drugs containing non-narcotic active medicinal ingredients. Any compound, mixture, or preparation containing any of the following narcotic drugs, or their salts calculated as the free anhydrous base or alkaloid, in limited quantities as set forth below, which must include one or more non-narcotic active medicinal ingredients in sufficient proportion to confer upon the compound, mixture, or preparation valuable medicinal qualities other than those possessed by narcotic drugs alone:

  (1) Not more than 200 milligrams of codeine per 100 milliliters or per 100 grams.

(2) Not more than 100 milligrams of dihydrocodeine per 100 milliliters or per 100 grams.

(3) Not more than 100 milligrams of ethylmorphine per 100 milliliters or per 100 grams.

(4) Not more than 2.5 milligrams of diphenoxylate and not less than 25 micrograms of atropine sulfate per dosage unit.

(5) Not more than 100 milligrams of opium per 100 milliliters or per 100 grams.

(6) Not more than 0.5 milligram of difenoxin and not less than 25 micrograms of atropine sulfate per dosage unit.

Study Tip

Note that all of the quantities listed above are evenly divisible by FIVE. This is a clue that they are classified in Schedule V.

Other specific examples of Schedule V products include

- Acetaminophen w/codeine elixir
- Promethazine w/codeine
- Diphenoxylate w/atropine (Lomotil)
- Ezogabine
- Lacosamide
- Pregabalin (Lyrica)

Excluded (Exempt) Substances

The following non-narcotic substances are some examples of drug products that contain controlled substances but are excluded or exempt from all schedules:

Brand Name	Controlled Substance Ingredient
Isuprel Elixir	Phenobarbital
Pyridium Plus Tablets	Butabarbital
Lufyllin-EPG Elixir	Phenobarbital
Butibel Tablets	Butabarbital sodium
Librax Caps	Chlordiazepoxide HCl
Donnatal Tabs and Elixir	Phenobarbital
Anaspaz PB	Phenobarbital

Note

Manufacturers may apply to the DEA for exemption of a product from controlled substance status. The exemption may be granted if it appears unlikely that the product can be abused. Because most of these brand name excluded products are of little therapeutic value, just about all of them have been removed from the market. The DEA always provides a current list of products that contain controlled substances but are exempt from all controlled substance schedules. The list may be found on line by the name **Exempt Prescription Products List**.

Purchasing or Transferring Schedule I or II Substances

An order form (DEA Form 222) or its electronic equivalent is required for each sale or transfer of a schedule I or II controlled substance.

Note

DEA Form 222 or its electronic equivalent is required for purchases, transfer of schedule I and II products from one pharmacy to another, returns to a supplier, etc. Its use is not required when such drug products are transferred from a central fill pharmacy to a retail pharmacy.

Order forms may be obtained only by persons who are registered to handle controlled substances listed in schedules I and II, and by persons who are registered to export such substances. Persons not registered to handle controlled substances listed in schedule I or II and persons registered only to import controlled substances listed in any schedule are not entitled to obtain order forms.

An order form or its electronic equivalent may be executed only on behalf of the registrant and only if his/her controlled substance registration has not expired or been revoked or suspended.

When an individual applies for a registration, the applicant may indicate on the application form that order forms are needed.

Order Forms (DEA Form 222) are issued in mailing envelopes containing either seven or fourteen forms, each form containing an original, a duplicate, and a triplicate copy (i.e., Copy 1, Copy 2, and Copy 3) (see Figure G-1).

Figure G-1
Parts of DEA Form 222

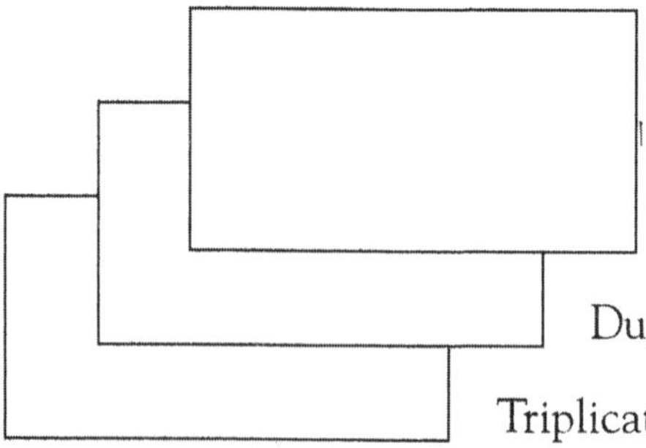

Original (Copy 1)
Duplicate (Copy 2)
Triplicate (Copy 3)

A limit, which is based on the business activity of the registrant, is imposed on the number of order forms that are furnished on any requisition unless additional forms are specifically requested and a reasonable need for such additional forms is shown. Additional forms may be requisitioned on the DEA Form 222a that is mailed to a registrant approximately 30 days after each shipment of order forms to that registrant. Registrants may also order additional forms by contacting any Division Office or the Registration Unit of the DEA.

All requisition forms (DEA Form 222a) must be submitted to the Registration Unit of the DEA. Each requisition must show the name, address, and registration number of the registrant and the number of books of order forms desired. Each requisition must be signed and dated by the same person who signed the most recent application for registration or for re-registration or by any person authorized to obtain and execute order forms by a Power of Attorney.

Order forms are serially numbered and issued with the name, address and registration number of the registrant, the authorized activity and schedules of the registrant. This information cannot be altered or changed by the registrant; the Registration Unit of the DEA must correct any errors by returning the forms with notification of the error.

Completing DEA Form 222

Order forms must be prepared and executed by the purchaser simultaneously in triplicate by means of interleaved carbon sheets that are part of the DEA Form 222 (see above). Order forms must be prepared by use of a typewriter, computer printer, pen, or indelible pencil.

Only one item may be entered on each numbered line of the order form. An item consists of one or more commercial or bulk containers of the same finished or bulk form and quantity of the same substance. The number of lines completed must be noted on that form at the bottom of the form, in the space provided.

> **Note**
>
> Remember that when ordering controlled substances on a DEA Form 222, a registrant is not permitted to order different drug products on the SAME LINE. For example, 3 x 100 Percodan tablets may be ordered on one line but NOT 1 x 100 Percodan and 1 x 100 codeine sulfate 30 mg tablets. Each different product must be ordered on a separate line.

The name and address of the supplier from whom the controlled substances are being ordered must be entered on the form. Only one supplier may be listed on any form.

Each order form must be signed and dated by a person authorized to sign an application for registration. The name of the purchaser, if different from the individual signing the order form, must also be inserted in the signature space.

Unexecuted order forms may be kept and may be executed at a location other than the registered location printed on the form. However, all unused forms must be promptly delivered to the registered site when any federal, state, or local inspector authorized to examine controlled substances, inspects the site.

Any purchaser may authorize one or more individuals to obtain and execute order forms on his/her behalf by creating a Power of Attorney for each such individual. The Power of Attorney must be signed by the same person who signed the most recent application for registration or re-registration and by the individual being given authorization to obtain and execute order forms. The Power of Attorney must be filed with the executed order forms of the purchaser, and must be retained for the same period as any order form bearing the signature of the Attorney. The Power of Attorney must be available for inspection together with other order form records.

Any Power of Attorney may be revoked at any time by executing a Notice of Revocation. This must be signed by the person who signed (or was authorized to sign) the Power of Attorney or by a successor, whoever signed the most recent application for registration or re-registration. It must be filed with the Power of Attorney being revoked. An example of the Power of Attorney form and notice of revocation is on following page.

Power of Attorney for DEA Order Forms and Electronic Orders

_________________________ (Name of registrant)

_________________________(Address of registrant)

_________________________(DEA registration number)

I, _________________ (name of person granting power), the undersigned, who am authorized to sign the current application for registration of the above-named registrant under the Controlled Substances Act or Controlled Substances Import and Export Act, do make, constitute, and appoint, and by these presents, do make, constitute, and appoint _________________________ (name of attorney-in-fact), my true and lawful attorney for me in my name, place, and stead, to execute applications for Forms 222 and to sign orders for Schedule I and II controlled substances, whether these orders be on Form 222 or electronic, in accordance with 21 U.S.C. 828 and Part 1305 of Title 21 of the Code of Federal Regulations. I hereby ratify and confirm all that said attorney shall lawfully do or cause to be done by virtue hereof _________________(Signature of person granting power)

I, ________ (name of attorney-in-fact), hereby affirm that I am the person named herein as attorney-in-fact and that the signature affixed hereto is my signature.

_________________________(Signature of attorney-in-fact)

Witnesses:

1. _________________. 2. _________________.

Signed and dated on the ______ day of __________, (year), at _________________.

Notice of Revocation

The foregoing power of attorney is hereby revoked by the undersigned, who is authorized to sign the current application for registration of the above-named registrant under the Controlled Substances Act of the Controlled Substances Import and Export Act. Written notice of this revocation has been given to the attorney-in-fact __________ this same day.

_________________________(Signature of person revoking power)

Witnesses: 1._________________2._________________

Signed and dated on the _______ day of __________, (year), at __________.

Filling Orders Written on DEA Form 222

Only a person registered as a manufacturer or distributor of controlled substances listed in Schedule I or II may fill an order form, except for the following:

- A pharmacist who is discontinuing a pharmacy.
- If a registrant's registration is expiring without re-registration.
- If a registrant is returning a Schedule I or II substance to the supplier (i.e. wholesaler or manufacturer) from which it was obtained.
- A person registered or authorized to conduct chemical analysis or research with controlled substances may distribute a controlled substance listed in Schedule I or II to another person registered or authorized to do the same.
- A person registered as a compounder of narcotic substances for use at off-site locations in conjunction with a narcotic treatment program at the compounding location. Such persons may fill orders for narcotic drugs for off-site narcotic treatment programs only.

> **Note**
>
> In summary, any transfer of Schedule I or II drugs from one registrant to another (e.g. pharmacy to pharmacy, pharmacy to wholesaler or manufacturer, etc.) requires the use of a DEA Form 222. Its use is not required when such drug products are transferred from a central fill pharmacy to a retail pharmacy.

Ordering Controlled Substances Using DEA Form 222

To order a controlled substance in Schedule I or II, the purchaser must complete DEA Form 222, submit Copy 1 and Copy 2 of the form to the supplier, and retain Copy 3 in his/her own files. The supplier fills the order, and records on Copies 1 and 2 the number of commercial or bulk containers furnished on each item and the date on which such containers are shipped to the purchaser.

If an order cannot be completely filled, it may be partially filled and the balance supplied by additional shipments within 60 days following the date of the order form. The order form is no longer valid after 60 days from the time it was executed by the purchaser.

The controlled substances may only be shipped to the purchaser and to the location printed by the DEA on the order form.

The supplier must retain Copy 1 of the order form for his/her own files and forward Copy 2, at the close of the month during which the order is filled, to the Special Agent in Charge of the DEA office in the area in which the supplier is located.

> **Study Tip**
>
> The supplier who fills a controlled substance order always keeps the original portion of the order. In this case, the supplier is "filling" the order for the purchaser. When a prescription is filled, the pharmacist is the supplier and, therefore, keeps the original prescription.

If a single order is filled by partial shipments, Copy 2 must be forwarded to the regional DEA office at the close of the month during which the final shipment is made or during which the 60-day validity period expires.

The purchaser (i.e. the pharmacist, physician, etc.) must record on Copy 3 of the order form the number of commercial or bulk containers received on each item and the dates on which such containers are received.

Study Tip

It is important to remember the colors and the final destination of each portion of DEA Form 222.

Copy 1 (Brown) - Goes to the supplier

Copy 2 (Green) - First goes to the supplier and is then forwarded to the DEA

Copy 3 (Blue) - Retained by the purchaser

Endorsing an Order Form

An order form made out to any supplier who cannot fill all or a part of the order within the specified time limitation may be endorsed to another supplier for filling.

The endorsement must be made only by the supplier to whom the order form was first made and must include (in the spaces provided on the reverse sides of Copies 1 and 2 of the order form)

- the name and address of the second supplier.
- the signature of a person authorized to obtain and execute order forms on behalf of the first supplier.

The first supplier may not fill any part of an order on an endorsed form. The second supplier must fill the order, if possible, and ship all substances directly to the purchaser.

Distributions made on endorsed order forms must be reported by the second supplier in the same manner as all other distributions except that where the name of the supplier is requested on the reporting form, the second supplier must record the name, address and registration number of the first supplier.

Unaccepted or Defective Order Forms

An order form must not be filled if it:

- is not complete, legible, or properly prepared, executed, or endorsed; or
- shows any alteration, erasure, or change of any description.

If an order cannot be filled for any reason, the supplier must return Copies 1 and 2 to the purchaser with a statement as to the reason (e.g., illegible, altered, etc.).

A supplier may for any reason refuse to accept any order. If a supplier refuses to accept the order, a statement that the order is not accepted is sufficient. When received by the purchaser, Copies 1 and 2 of the order form and the statement indicating why it was not filled must be attached to Copy 3 and retained in the files of the purchaser.

An order form that is incorrect may not be corrected. In order for the order to be filled, a new order form must replace it.

Lost or Stolen Order Forms

If a purchaser determines that an unfilled order form has been lost, he/she must prepare another form in triplicate. The purchaser must also prepare a statement containing the serial number and date of the lost form. The statement should indicate that the goods covered by the first order form were not received because that order form was lost.

Copy 3 of the second form and a copy of the statement must be retained with Copy 3 of the order form first executed. A copy of the statement must be attached to Copies 1 and 2 of the second order form sent to the supplier. If the supplier to whom the order was directed subsequently receives the first order form, the supplier must write "Not accepted" on the face of the form and return Copies 1 and 2 to the purchaser, who must attach it to Copy 3 and the statement.

Whenever any used or unused order forms are stolen or lost (other than in the course of transmission) by any purchaser or supplier, he/she must immediately report the loss to the Special Agent in Charge of the DEA in the Divisional Office responsible for the area in which the registrant is located. The report must state the serial number of each form stolen or lost. If the theft or loss includes any original order forms received from purchasers and the supplier is unable to state the serial numbers of such order forms, he/she must report the date or approximate date of receipt thereof and the names and addresses of the purchasers.

If an entire book of order forms is lost or stolen, and the purchaser is unable to state the serial numbers of the lost order forms, he/she must report the date or approximate date of issuance of the forms instead. If any unused order form reported stolen or lost is subsequently recovered or found, the Special Agent in Charge of the DEA in the Divisional Office responsible for the area in which the registrant is located must immediately be notified.

Study Tip

Carefully review the process of ordering Schedule I and II drugs. An excellent way to review this process is to prepare a simulated, triplicate DEA Form 222 and practice the ordering process, perhaps using a friend as the "supplier".

Storage of Order Forms

The PURCHASER must retain Copy 3 of each order form that has been filled. He/she must also retain in his/her files all copies of each unaccepted or defective order form and each statement attached thereto. Order forms must be maintained separately from all other records of the Registrant.

The SUPPLIER must retain Copy 1 of each order form that he/she has filled.

Order forms and other related documents must be kept available for inspection for a period of two years.

A supplier of carfentanil, etorphine hydrochloride and diprenorphine must maintain order forms for these substances separately from all other order forms and records.

> ***Note***
>
> Carfentanil and etorphine hydrochloride are potent narcotics that are used exclusively in veterinary practice. They are often used to immobilize large animals. Diprenorphine is an opioid antagonist used to reverse the effects of these two narcotic agents.

Return of Unused Order Forms

If the registration of any purchaser terminates (because the purchaser dies, ceases legal existence, discontinues business or professional practice), or changes the name or address as shown on his registration, or if his/her registration is suspended or revoked, all unused order forms must be returned to the nearest office of the DEA.

Cancellation and Voiding of Order Forms

A purchaser may cancel part or all of an order on an order form by notifying the supplier in writing of such cancellation. The supplier must indicate the cancellation on Copies 1 and 2 of the order form by drawing a line through the cancelled items and printing "canceled' in the space provided for number of items shipped.

A supplier may void part or all of an order on an order form by notifying the purchaser in writing of such voiding. The supplier must indicate the voiding in the manner prescribed for cancellation in the previous paragraph.

Controlled Substance Ordering System (CSOS)

The Controlled Substances Ordering System (CSOS) provides an electronic equivalent to the DEA official order form (Form 222). CSOS regulations permit, but does not require, registrants to order Schedule I and II substances electronically and maintain the records of these orders electronically.

The advantages of electronic ordering include

- Greater Ordering Freedom: CSOS transactions are the only allowance for electronic ordering of Schedule I and II controlled substances, but may also be used for Schedule III-V substances. Additionally, unlike the paper Form 222, which is limited to ordering a maximum of ten items per form, CSOS has no line item limit for a single order.
- Faster Transactions: CSOS certificates contain the same identification information as DEA Form 222, which allows for timely and accurate validation by the supplier. Faster transactions allow for rapid ordering and smaller inventories.
- Accurate Orders: CSOS reduces the number of ordering errors.
- Decreased Cost: Order accuracy and decreased paper work result in a lower transaction cost.

Note

As of September, 2016 the Drug Enforcement Administration (DEA) will have advised all DEA registrants of changes in communicating to DEA's Office of Diversion Control websites. All registrants will be required to upgrade their browsers and systems to support Transport Layer Security (TLS) version 1.2 or higher. This is designed to provide greater protection of data transmitted to and from DEA.

Enrollment in CSOS

To enroll in CSOS, the individual purchaser is required to acquire a CSOS digital certificate. Using a technology called Public Key Infrastructure (PKI), a Certification Authority verifies the identity of applicants before issuing digital certificates and public-private key pairs to them. The holder of the digital certificate has a private key, which only the certificate holder can access, and a public key, which is available to anyone. What one key encrypts, only the other key can decrypt. Only one public key will validate signatures made using its corresponding private key. Because only one person holds the private key, it is that person's responsibility to ensure that it is not divulged or compromised.

Purchaser Requirements

- To be a valid order, the purchaser must sign an electronic order for a Schedule I or II controlled substance with a digital signature issued to the purchaser, or the purchaser's agent, by the DEA.
- The following data fields must be included on an electronic order for Schedule I and II controlled substances:

  (1) A unique number the purchaser assigns to track the order.

The number must be in the following 9-character format: the last two digits of the year, X, and six characters as selected by the purchaser.

(e.g. 10X123456)

(2) The purchaser's DEA registration number.

(3) The name of the supplier.

(4) The complete address of the supplier (may be completed by either the purchaser or the supplier).

(5) The supplier's DEA registration number (may be completed by either the purchaser or the supplier).

(6) The date the order is signed.

(7) The name (including strength where appropriate) of the controlled substance product or the National Drug Code (NDC) number (the NDC number may be completed by either the purchaser or the supplier).

(8) The quantity in a single package or container.

(9) The number of packages or containers of each item ordered.

- An electronic order may include controlled substances that are not in schedules I and II and may also include non-controlled substances.

> **Note**
>
> Notice that electronic orders may include items that are in any controlled substance categories as well as non-controlled substances.

Supplier Requirements

Before filling an electronic order, the supplier must

— verify the integrity of the signature and the order by using software that complies with CSOS regulations.

— verify that the digital certificate has not expired.

— check the validity of the certificate holder's certificate by checking the Certificate Revocation List.

- The supplier must retain an electronic record of every order, and, linked to each order, a record of the number of commercial or bulk containers furnished on each item and the date on which the supplier shipped the containers to the purchaser. The linked record must also include any data on the original order that the supplier completes.
- If an order cannot be filled in its entirety, a supplier may fill it in part and supply the balance by additional shipments within 60 days following the date of the order.
- No order is valid more than 60 days after its execution by the purchaser.
- A supplier must ship the controlled substances to the registered location associated with the digital certificate used to sign the order.

When a purchaser receives a shipment, the purchaser must create a record of the quantity of each item received and the date received. The record must be electronically linked to the original order and archived.

- A supplier may not endorse an electronic order to another supplier to fill.
- A supplier must, for each electronic order filled, forward either a copy of the electronic order or an electronic report of the order, in a format that DEA specifies, to DEA within two business days.

Invalid Orders

- No electronic order may be filled if:

(1) the required data fields have not been completed.

(2) the order is not signed using a digital certificate issued by DEA.

(3) the digital certificate used has expired or has been revoked prior to signature.

(4) the purchaser's public key will not validate the digital signature.

(5) the validation of the order shows that the order is invalid for any reason.

- If an order cannot be filled for any reason, the supplier must notify the purchaser and provide a statement as to the reason (e.g., if the order has been improperly prepared or altered). A supplier may, for any reason, refuse to accept any order and, if a supplier refuses to accept the order, a statement that the order is not accepted is sufficient notification.

- When a purchaser receives an unaccepted electronic order from the supplier, the purchaser must electronically link the statement of nonacceptance to the original order. The original order and the statement must be retained.

- Neither a purchaser or a supplier may correct a defective order; the purchaser must issue a new order for the order to be filled.

Lost Orders

- If a purchaser determines that an unfilled electronic order has been lost before or after receipt, the purchaser must provide, to the supplier, a signed statement containing the unique tracking number and date of the lost order and stating that the goods covered by the first order were not received through loss of that order.

- If the purchaser executes an order to replace the lost order, the purchaser must electronically link an electronic record of the second order and a copy of the statement with the record of the first order and retain them.

- If the supplier to whom the order was directed subsequently receives the first order, the supplier must indicate that it is "Not Accepted" and return it to the purchaser. The purchaser must link the returned order to the record of that order and the statement.
- A purchaser must, for each order filled, retain the original signed order and all linked records for that order for two years. The purchaser must also retain all copies of each unaccepted or defective order and each linked statement.
- A supplier must retain each original order filled and the linked records for two years.
- If electronic order records are maintained on a central server, the records must be readily retrievable at the registered location.

Canceling and Voiding Electronic Orders

- A supplier may void all or part of an electronic order by notifying the purchaser of the voiding. If the entire order is voided, the supplier must make an electronic copy of the order, indicate on the copy "Void", and return it to the purchaser. The supplier is not required to retain a record of orders that are not filled.
- The purchaser must retain an electronic copy of the voided order.
- To partially void an order, the supplier must indicate in the linked record that nothing was shipped for each item voided.

Compounding or Repackaging With Controlled Substances

If a registrant purchases a controlled substance for the purpose of repackaging them for sale within the pharmacy or to other registrants, the registrant must register as a manufacturer.

A pharmacist may compound controlled substances for "office use" as long as the product

- is compounded as an aqueous, oleaginous or solid dosage form.
- does not contain more than 20% controlled substance.
- is only distributed to a practitioner who is authorized to dispense.

Persons Entitled To Issue Controlled Substance Prescriptions

A prescription for a controlled substance may be issued only by an individual practitioner who is:

- authorized to prescribe controlled substances by the jurisdiction in which he/she is licensed to practice his profession, and
- either registered or exempted from registration pursuant to the CSA.

An employee or agent of the individual practitioner (e.g. a nurse, secretary) may communicate a prescription issued by an individual practitioner to a pharmacist.

Purpose for Issuing of Controlled Substances Prescriptions

- In order to be a valid controlled substance prescription, an individual practitioner, acting in the usual course of their professional practice, must issue the prescription for a legitimate medical purpose.
- The responsibility for the proper prescribing and dispensing of controlled substances is upon the prescribing practitioner, but a corresponding responsibility rests with the pharmacist who

fills the prescription.

- An order/prescription that is not issued in the usual course of professional treatment or as part of legitimate and authorized research is not a prescription. A person knowingly filling such an order or prescription, as well as the person issuing it, is in violation of the CSA.

A prescription may not be issued for an individual practitioner to obtain controlled substances for the purpose of general dispensing to patients.

> **Note**
>
> If a practitioner wishes to dispense controlled substances to patients, he/she must order them directly from a supplier (i.e. a wholesaler or manufacturer). In other words, prescribing controlled substances for "office use" is not permissible.

A prescription may not be issued for "detoxification treatment" or "maintenance treatment," unless the prescription is for a Schedule III, IV, or V narcotic drug approved by the Food and Drug Administration specifically for use in maintenance or detoxification treatment and the practitioner is in compliance with requirements specified in the CSA.

Practitioner Self-prescribing

Under federal law, a controlled substance prescription is valid only if it is "issued for a legitimate medical purpose by a practitioner acting in the usual course of sound professional practice." While federal law is not specific with regard to self-prescribing, Policy E-8.19 of the American Medical Association (AMA) states: "Physicians should generally not treat themselves or members of their immediate family," and makes an exception only for certain emergency situations.

It is the responsibility of prescribers to use good professional judgement and it is the legal responsibility of the pharmacist to adhere to sound professional practice in filling prescriptions. What constitutes "sound professional practice" is left to state laws.

Issuing Of Controlled Substance Prescriptions

- All prescriptions for controlled substances must be dated and signed on the day when written and must bear the:
  - full name and address of the patient.
  - drug name, strength, and dosage form.
  - quantity prescribed.
  - directions for use.
  - name, address and registration number (i.e. DEA number) of the practitioner.
- A prescription for a Schedule III, IV, or V narcotic drug approved by FDA specifically for "detoxification treatment" or "maintenance treatment" must include the identification number issued to the practitioner by the DEA Administrator.
- A practitioner must sign a prescription in the same manner as he/she would sign a check or legal document (e.g., J.H. Smith or John H. Smith).
- Where an oral order is not permitted, paper prescriptions must be written with ink or indelible pencil, typewriter, or printed on a computer and must be manually signed by practitioner. A computer-generated prescription that is printed out or faxed by the practitioner must be manually signed.
- An agent of the practitioner (e.g. a secretary or nurse) may prepare prescriptions for the practitioner's signature, but the prescribing practitioner is still responsible for assuring that the prescription conforms in all essential respects to the law and regulations. A corresponding liability rests upon the pharma-

cist who fills a prescription that is prepared in proper form.

- An individual practitioner exempted from registration under the CSA must instead include on all prescriptions issued by him or her, the registration number of the hospital or other institution and the special internal code number assigned to him or her by the hospital or other institution.

Study Tip

In studying the laws that pertain to the creation and dispensing of controlled substances it is essential to review your state requirements. Many have their own requirements for these drugs.

Note

Many states permit institutions such as hospitals to provide institutional prescribers who do not have their own registration number with the hospital DEA number plus a numerical suffix that specifically identifies the prescriber.

Each written prescription must have the name of the physician stamped, typed, or hand-printed on it, as well as the signature of the physician.

- An official exempted from registration under the CSA (e.g. a military or Public Health Service physician) must include his/her branch of service or agency (e.g., "U.S. Army" or "Public Health Service") and service identification number on all prescriptions issued, instead of the DEA number usually required.

The service identification number for a Public Health Service employee is his/her Social Security number. Each prescription must have the name of the officer stamped, typed, or hand-printed on it, as well as the signature of the officer.

Persons Entitled To Fill Controlled Substance Prescriptions

Only a pharmacist, acting in the usual course of his/her professional practice, may fill a prescription for controlled substances. Such a pharmacist must either be registered individually or employed in a registered pharmacy or registered institutional pharmacy.

Electronic Prescriptions for Controlled Substances

The DEA provides practitioners with the option of writing prescriptions for controlled substances electronically. It also permits pharmacies to receive, dispense, and archive these electronic prescriptions.

These regulations do not mandate that practitioners prescribe controlled substances using only electronic prescriptions. Nor do they require pharmacies to accept electronic prescriptions for controlled substances for dispensing. Whether a practitioner or pharmacy uses electronic prescriptions for controlled substances is voluntary from DEA's perspective. Prescribing practitioners are still able to write, and manually sign, prescriptions for schedule II, III, IV, and V controlled substances and pharmacies are still able to dispense controlled substances based on those written prescriptions. Oral prescriptions remain valid for schedule III, IV, and V controlled substances.

Certification

The provider of the application (e.g. a computer program) to be used by a pharmacy or practitioner must either hire a qualified third party to audit the application or have the application reviewed and certified by an approved certification body. The auditor or certification body will issue a report that states whether the application complies with DEA's requirements and whether there are any limitations on its use for controlled substance prescriptions. (A limited set of prescriptions require information that may need revision of the basic prescription standard before they can be reliably accommodated.) The application provider must provide a copy of the report to practitioners or pharmacies to allow them to determine whether the application is compliant.

Identity Proofing

Identity proofing is required in order to utilize electronic prescribing of controlled substances. Authorization to prescribe will not be granted to a practitioner until their identity has been confirmed. Individual practitioners must obtain two-factor authentication credential or digital certificates from federally approved credential service providers (CSPs) or certification authorities (CAs). For two-factor authorization, DEA will permit the use of two of the following

- something you know (a knowledge factor)
- something you have (a hard token stored separately from the computer being accessed), and
- something you are (biometric information).

The hard token, if used, must be a cryptographic device or a one-time-password device that meets Federal Information Processing standards.

The practitioner must use the two-factor credential to sign the prescription; that is, using the two-factor credential constitutes the legal signature of the DEA-registered prescribing practitioner. When the credential is used, the application must digitally sign and archive at least the DEA-required information contained in the prescription.

An agent of the practitioner may enter information at the practitioner's direction prior to the practitioner reviewing and approving the information as long as the practitioner signs and authorizes the transmission of the prescription. In addition, the practitioner is responsible in the event the prescription does not conform in all essential respects to the law and regulations.

Prescription Copies

A practitioner may print copies of any electronic prescriptions for controlled substances if they are clearly labeled: "Copy only – not valid for dispensing." Data on the prescription may be electronically transferred to medical records, and a list of prescriptions transmitted may be printed for patients if the list indicates that it is for informational purposes only and not for dispensing. The copies must be printed **after** transmission. If an electronic prescription is printed prior to attempted transmission, the electronic prescription application must not allow it to be transmitted.

Multiple Patients and Prescriptions

A practitioner is not permitted to issue prescriptions for multiple patients with a single signature. However, a practitioner is allowed to sign multiple prescriptions for a single patient at one time. Each controlled substance prescription will have to be indicated as ready for signing, but a single execution of the two-factor authentication protocol can then sign all prescriptions for a given patient that the practitioner has indicated as being ready to be signed.

Once an electronic controlled substance prescription is signed, it does not need to be transmitted to the pharmacy immediately. Signing and transmitting an electronic controlled substance prescription are two distinct actions. Electronic prescriptions for controlled substances should be transmitted as soon as possible after signing. However, it is understood that practitioners may prefer to sign prescriptions before office staff add pharmacy or insurance information. Therefore, DEA does not requiring that transmission of the prescription occur simultaneously with signing the prescription.

Transmission Failure

If transmission of an electronic prescription fails, the electronic prescription may not be converted by an intermediary to another form (e.g. facsimile) for transmission. An electronic prescription must be transmitted from the practitioner to the pharmacy in its electronic form. If an intermediary cannot complete a transmission of a controlled substance prescription, the intermediary must notify the practitioner. Under such circumstances, if the prescription is for a schedule III, IV, or V controlled substance, the practitioner can print the prescription, manually sign it, and fax the prescription directly to the pharmacy. This prescription must indicate that it was originally transmitted to, and provide the name of, a specific pharmacy, the date and time of transmission, and the fact that the electronic transmission failed.

Prescription Alterations

An electronic prescription may not be altered as it is transmitted from a practitioner to a pharmacy. This does not apply to changes that occur after receipt at the pharmacy. Changes made by the pharmacy are governed by the same laws and regulations that apply to paper prescriptions.

Prescription Back-up

Pharmacy application service providers must back-up files daily. Also, although it is not required, DEA recommends as a best practice that pharmacies store their back-up copies at another location to prevent the loss of the records in the event of natural disasters, fires, or system failures.

Once a prescription is created electronically, all records of the prescription must be retained electronically. As is the case with paper prescription records, electronic controlled substance prescription records must be kept for a minimum period of two years.

Duplicate Prescriptions

If pharmacist receives a paper or oral prescription that was originally transmitted electronically to the pharmacy, the pharmacist must check the pharmacy records to ensure that the electronic version was not received and the prescription dispensed. If both prescriptions were received, the pharmacist must mark one as void. If a pharmacist receives a paper or oral prescription that indicates that it was originally transmitted electronically to another pharmacy, the pharmacist must check with the other pharmacy to determine whether the prescription was received and dispensed. If the pharmacy that received the original electronic prescription has not dispensed the prescription, that pharmacy must mark the electronic version as void or canceled. If the pharmacy that received the original electronic prescription dispensed the prescription, the pharmacy with the paper version must not dispense the paper prescription and must mark the prescription as void.

Detoxification or Maintenance Treatment

In order to administer or dispense (but not prescribe) narcotic drugs listed in any schedule to a narcotic drug-dependent person for "detoxification treatment" or "maintenance treatment" a practitioner must be separately registered with DEA and must comply with the special regulatory standards imposed relative to treatment qualification, security, records and unsupervised use of drugs.

A physician who is not specifically registered to conduct a narcotic treatment program may administer (but not prescribe) narcotic drugs to a person for the purpose of relieving acute withdrawal symptoms, when necessary, while arrangements are being made for referral for treatment. Not more than one day's medication may be administered to the person or for the person's use at one time. Such emergency treatment may be carried out for not more than three days and may not be renewed or extended.

Schedule II Prescription Requirements

Written Prescriptions and Orders

A pharmacist may normally dispense a Schedule II controlled substance prescription drug pursuant to a written prescription signed by the practitioner. A pharmacist may also dispense a controlled substance pursuant to an electronic order under the guidelines discussed in the previous section.

An individual practitioner may administer or dispense directly a Schedule II controlled substance in the course of his/her professional practice without a prescription to a narcotic dependant person for the purpose of maintenance or detoxification treatment if the practitioner meets both of the following conditions:

(1) The practitioner is separately registered with DEA as a narcotic treatment program.

(2) The practitioner is in compliance with DEA regulations regarding treatment qualifications, security, records, and unsupervised use of the drugs pursuant to the CSA.

A physician who is not specifically registered to conduct a narcotic treatment program may administer, but not prescribe, narcotic drugs to a person for the purpose of relieving acute withdrawal symptoms when necessary while arrangements are being made for referral for treatment. Not more than one day's medication may be administered to the person or for the person's use at one time. Such emergency treatment may be carried out for not more than three days and may not be renewed or extended.

An institutional practitioner may administer or dispense directly (but not prescribe):

- a Schedule II controlled substance pursuant to a written prescription signed by the prescribing practitioner; or
- an order for Schedule II medication that is to be dispensed for immediate administration to the ultimate user.

Oral Prescriptions or Orders

In an emergency situation, a pharmacist may dispense a Schedule II controlled substance upon receiving the oral authorization of a prescribing practitioner, provided that:

- the quantity prescribed and dispensed is limited to the amount adequate to treat the patient during the emergency period (dispensing beyond the emergency period must be pursuant to a written prescription signed by the prescribing practitioner).
- the prescription must be immediately reduced to writing by the pharmacist and must contain all required information except for the signature of the prescriber.
- if the pharmacist does not know the prescriber, he/she must make a reasonable effort to determine that the oral order is legitimate. Such effort(s) may include a callback to the prescriber using his/her phone number as listed in the telephone directory and/or other good faith efforts to insure his/her identity.
- within seven (7) days after authorizing an emergency oral prescription, the prescriber must have delivered to the dispensing pharmacist a written prescription for the emergency quantity prescribed. In addition to conforming to the usual requirements for written Schedule II drug prescriptions, this "cover" prescription must have written on its face "Authorization for Emergency Dispensing," and the date of the oral order. The "cover" prescription may be delivered to the pharmacist in person or by mail. If it is delivered by mail it must be postmarked within the seven-day period. Upon receipt of the "cover" prescription, the dispensing pharmacist is required to attach this prescription to the oral emergency prescription that had earlier been reduced to writing.

The pharmacist is required to notify the nearest DEA office if the prescriber fails to deliver a written "cover" prescription to him/her in a timely basis.

Central fill pharmacies are not permitted to prepare prescriptions for a controlled substance listed in Schedule II upon receiving an oral authorization from a retail pharmacist or an individual practitioner.

What Is An Emergency?

For the purposes of authorizing an oral prescription of a controlled substance listed in Schedule II, the term "emergency situation" means those situations in which the prescriber determines that:

- immediate administration of the controlled substance is necessary for proper treatment of the intended ultimate user; and
- no appropriate alternative treatment is available, including administration of a drug which is not a schedule II controlled substance; and
- it is not reasonably possible for the prescriber to provide a written prescription to be presented to the person dispensing the substance, prior to the dispensing.

Missing Information

Over the past decade the DEA has provided mixed messages with regard to a pharmacist making additions or changes to written Schedule II prescriptions. To date, the DEA has instructed pharmacists to adhere to state regulations or policy regarding those changes that a pharmacist may make to a schedule II prescription after oral consultation with the prescriber. Therefore, when information is missing from or needs to be changed on a schedule II controlled substance prescription, DEA expects pharmacists to use their professional judgment and knowledge of state and federal laws and policies to decide whether it is appropriate to make changes to that prescription.

Of course, a pharmacist is never permitted to make changes in the patient's name, the controlled substance prescribed (except generic substitution permitted by state law), or the prescriber's signature. If any of these items must be changed, a new prescription is required from the prescriber.

Faxing of Schedule II Prescriptions

Faxing of a Schedule II prescription to the dispensing pharmacy by the prescriber or the prescriber's agent is permitted for:

- home infusion pharmacies receiving prescriptions intended for parenteral administration.
- a resident of a Long Term Care Facility (LTCF).
- schedule II controlled substance prescriptions, written for a patient enrolled in hospice, certified by or licensed by the state may be faxed to a pharmacy for dispensing. The hospice patient may reside in a personal residence or hospice facility. The practitioner or the practitioner's agent must note on the prescription that the patient is a hospice patient.

In each case, the fax serves as the original written prescription and must be filed accordingly.

In all other cases, a prescription order for a Schedule II drug product may only be faxed for information purposes and may not serve as the original prescription order. The prescription may only be dispensed once the original is presented.

> **Note**
>
> Many states have their own regulations pertaining to faxing of controlled substances. Be sure to check on these before taking the licensing examination.

Refilling Schedule II Prescriptions

The refilling of Schedule II prescriptions is prohibited.

Partial Filling of Schedule II Prescriptions

The partial filling of Schedule II controlled substance prescriptions is permissible. If the pharmacist is unable to supply the full quantity called for in a written or emergency oral prescription, he/she must make a notation of the quantity supplied on the face of the written prescription (or written record of the emergency oral prescription). The remaining portion of the prescription may be filled within 72 hours of the first partial filling. If the remaining portion is not or cannot be filled within the 72-hour period, the pharmacist must notify the prescribing individual practitioner. No further quantity may be supplied beyond 72 hours without a new prescription.

Note

Partial filling of a Schedule II prescription is not permitted if it is being done on the request of the patient (e.g. if a patient only wants half of the medication the prescription calls for). Partial filling is only permitted if the pharmacist is unable to supply the full quantity prescribed (e.g. because he/she is out of stock).

A prescription for a Schedule II controlled substance written for a patient in a Long Term Care Facility (LTCF) or for a patient with a medical diagnosis documenting a terminal illness may be filled in partial quantities. If there is any question as to whether a patient may be classified as having a terminal illness, the pharmacist must contact the prescriber prior to partially filling the prescription. Both the pharmacist and the prescriber have a corresponding responsibility to assure that the controlled substance is for a terminally ill patient. The pharmacist must record on the prescription whether the patient is "terminally ill"' or an "LTCF patient". A prescription that is partially filled and does not contain one of these designations is assumed to have been filled in violation of the CSA.

For each partial filling, the dispensing pharmacist must record on the BACK of the prescription (or on another appropriate record, uniformly maintained, and readily retrievable) the

- date of the partial filling.
- quantity dispensed.
- remaining quantity authorized to be dispensed.
- identification of the dispensing pharmacist.

The total quantity of Schedule II controlled substances dispensed in all partial fillings is not permitted to exceed the total quantity prescribed.

Schedule II prescriptions for patients in a LTCF or patients with a medical diagnosis documenting a terminal illness are valid for a period not to exceed 60 days from the issue date.

Information related to current Schedule II prescriptions for patients in a LTCF or for patients with a medical diagnosis documenting a terminal illness may be maintained in a computerized system if this system has the capability to permit:

- output (display or printout) of the original prescription number, date of issue, identification of prescribing individual practitioner, identification of patient, address of the LTCF or address of the hospital or residence of the patient, identification of medication authorized (to include dosage, form, strength and quantity), listing of the partial fillings that have been dispensed under each prescription and other information required by the CSA.
- immediate (real time) updating of the prescription record each time a partial filling of the prescription is conducted.

Labeling Schedule II Prescriptions

The pharmacist filling a written or emergency oral prescription for a Schedule II controlled substance must affix to the prescription package a label showing the

- date of filling
- pharmacy name and address
- serial number of the prescription
- name of the patient
- name of the prescribing practitioner
- directions for use
- following warning: "Caution: Federal law prohibits the transfer of this drug to any person other than the patient for whom it was prescribed."

> **Note**
>
> This "Caution" statement is not required to appear on the label of a Schedule II controlled substance dispensed for use in clinical investigations which are "blinded" (e.g. a double-blinded study).

- other cautionary statements, if any, contained in such prescription or required by law.

> **Note**
>
> If the prescription is filled at a central fill pharmacy, the central fill pharmacy must affix to the package a label showing the retail pharmacy name and address and a unique identifier, (i.e. the central fill pharmacy's DEA registration number) indicating that the prescription was filled at the central fill pharmacy, in addition to the information listed above.

These requirements do not apply when a controlled substance

listed in Schedule II is prescribed for administration to a patient in an institution, provided that:

- not more than 7-day supply of the Schedule II controlled substance is dispensed at one time.
- the controlled substance listed in Schedule II is not in the possession of the ultimate user prior to the administration.
- the institution maintains appropriate safeguards and records regarding the proper administration, control, dispensing, and storage of the controlled substance listed in Schedule II, and
- the system employed by the pharmacist in filling a prescription is adequate to identify the supplier, the product, and the patient, and to set forth the directions for use and cautionary statements, if any, contained in the prescription or required by law.

Schedule III, IV, and V Prescription Requirements

A pharmacist may dispense a Schedule III, IV, or V controlled substance prescription drug only pursuant to

- a written prescription signed by a practitioner, or
- a fax of a written, signed prescription transmitted by the prescriber or the prescriber's agent to the pharmacy, or
- an electronic prescription that meets CSA requirements
- an oral prescription made by an individual practitioner and promptly reduced to writing by the pharmacist containing all information required except for the signature of the prescriber.

A prescriber may administer or dispense a Schedule III, IV, or V controlled substance directly to a consumer in the course of their professional practice without a prescription.

An institutional practitioner-pharmacist may administer or dispense directly (but not prescribe) a Schedule III, IV, or V controlled substance only pursuant to

- a written prescription signed by a prescriber.
- a fax of a written prescription or order for medication transmitted by the prescriber or the prescriber's agent to the institutional practitioner-pharmacist.
- an electronic prescription that meets the requirements of the CSA.
- an oral prescription made by a prescriber and promptly reduced to writing by the pharmacist (containing all required information except for the signature of the prescriber).
- an order for medication made by a prescriber which is dispensed for immediate administration to the ultimate user.

Refilling of Schedule III, IV or V Prescriptions

Prescriptions for Schedule III or IV controlled substances may be refilled not more than five times in a six-month period from the date on which such prescription was issued, if authorized by the prescriber. Written Schedule V prescriptions may be refilled in accordance with the prescriber's instructions.

> **Note**
>
> Many states limit refills of Schedule V prescriptions to the same maximum of five refills within a six-month period.

A record of each refilling of a prescription must be entered on the back of the prescription or on another appropriate document or electronic prescription record. If entered on another document, such as a medication record or electronic prescription record, the document or record must be uniformly maintained and readily retrievable. The following information must be retrievable by the prescription number:

- Name and dosage form of the controlled substance
- Date filled or refilled
- Quantity dispensed
- Initials of the dispensing pharmacist for each refill
- The total number of refills for that prescription

If the pharmacist just initials and dates the back of the prescription or annotates the electronic prescription record it is assumed that the full amount of the prescription has been dispensed as a refill.

The prescribing practitioner may authorize additional refills of Schedule III or IV controlled substances on the original prescription through an oral refill authorization transmitted to the pharmacist provided the following conditions are met:

- The total quantity authorized, including the amount of the original prescription, does not exceed five refills within a six-month period from the date of issue of the original prescription.
- The pharmacist obtaining the oral authorization must record on the reverse of the original paper prescription or annotates the electronic prescription record
  - — the date of authorization.
  - — the quantity of medication per refill.
  - — the number of additional refills authorized.
  - — his/her initials on the paper prescription or annotates the electronic prescription record showing who received the authorization from the prescribing practitioner who issued the original prescription.
- The quantity of each additional refill authorized is equal to or less than the quantity authorized for the initial filling of the original prescription.
- The prescriber must issue a new and separate prescription for any additional quantities beyond the five refills, six-month

limitation.

As an alternative to the procedures described above, a computer application may be used for the storage and retrieval of refill information for prescription orders for Schedule III and IV controlled substances, subject to the following conditions:

- The computerized application must provide on-line retrieval (via computer monitor or hard-copy printout) of original prescription order information for those prescription orders, which are currently authorized for refilling. This must include, but is not limited to the:
  - — original prescription number.
  - — date of issuance of the original prescription order by the prescriber.
  - — full name and address of the patient.
  - — name, address, and DEA registration number of the prescriber.
  - — name, strength, dosage form and quantity of the controlled substance prescribed (and quantity dispensed if different from the quantity prescribed).
  - — total number of refills authorized by the prescriber.
- The computerized application must provide on-line retrieval (via computer monitor or hard-copy printout) of the current refill history for Schedule III or IV controlled substance prescription orders (those authorized for refill during the past six months.) This refill history must include, but is not limited to the
  - — name of the controlled substance.
  - — date of refill.
  - — quantity dispensed.
  - — identification code, or name or initials of the dispensing pharmacist for each refill.
  - — total number of refills dispensed to date for that prescrip-

tion order.

- The individual pharmacist who makes use of such a system must provide documentation of the fact that the refill information entered into the computer for a Schedule III or IV controlled substance is correct.

- If such a system provides a hard-copy printout of each day's controlled substance prescription order refill data, that printout must be verified, dated, and signed by the individual pharmacist who refilled such a prescription order. The individual pharmacist must verify that the data indicated is correct and then sign this document in the same manner as he/she would sign a check or legal document (e.g., C. H. Smith, or Chris H. Smith). This document must be maintained in a separate file at that pharmacy for a period of two years from the dispensing date. This printout of the day's controlled substance prescription order refill data must be provided to each pharmacy using such a computerized system within 72 hours of the date on which the refill was dispensed. It must be verified and signed by each pharmacist who is involved with such dispensing. In lieu of such a printout, the pharmacy must maintain a bound log book, or separate file, in which each individual pharmacist involved in such dispensing must sign a statement each day. The statement must attest to the fact that the refill information entered into the computer that day has been reviewed by him/her and is correct as shown. Such a book or file must be maintained at the pharmacy using such a system for a period of two years after the date of dispensing the appropriately authorized refill.

- Any such computerized application must have the capability of producing a printout of any refill data that the user pharmacy is responsible for maintaining under the CSA. For example, this would include a refill-by-refill audit trail for any specified strength and dosage form of any controlled substance (by either brand or generic name or both). Such a printout must include the

— name of the prescriber.

— name and address of the patient.

— quantity dispensed on each refill.

— date of dispensing for each refill.

— name or identification code of the dispensing pharmacist.

— number of the original prescription order.

- In any computerized application employed by a user pharmacy, the central recordkeeping location must be capable of sending the printout to the pharmacy within 48 hours.
- In the event that a pharmacy employing such a computerized application experiences system downtime, the pharmacy must have an auxiliary procedure which will be used for documenting refills of Schedule III and IV controlled substance prescription orders. This auxiliary procedure must insure that refills are authorized by the original prescription order, that the maximum number of refills has not been exceeded, and that all of the appropriate data is retained for on-line data entry as soon as the computer system is available for use again.

Note

When filing refill information for original prescription orders for Schedule III or IV controlled substances, a pharmacy may use only one of the two systems described above (i.e. putting the information on the back of the original prescription or onto a computerized record-keeping system).

Partial Filling of Schedule III, IV, and V Prescriptions

The partial filling of a prescription for a controlled substance listed in Schedule III, IV, or V is permissible, provided that:

- each partial filling is recorded in the same manner as a refill (see above).
- the total quantity dispensed in all partial fillings does not exceed the total quantity prescribed.
- no dispensing occurs beyond 6 months after the date on which the prescription was issued.

Labeling and Filling of Schedule III, IV and V Prescriptions

The pharmacist filling a prescription for a Schedule III, IV, or V controlled substance must affix to the package a label showing the

- pharmacy name and address.
- serial number.
- date of initial filling.
- name of the patient.
- name of the practitioner issuing the prescription.
- directions for use.

> ### Note
>
> Remember that the warning: "Caution: Federal law prohibits the transfer of this drug to any person other than the patient for whom it was prescribed" must also be applied to the prescription container of Schedule II, III and IV prescriptions except those that are for use in clinical investigations, which are "blinded".

- cautionary statements, if any, contained in the prescription, as required by law.

If the prescription is filled at a central fill pharmacy, the central fill pharmacy must affix to the package a label showing the retail pharmacy name and address and a unique identifier, (i.e. the central fill pharmacy's DEA registration number) indicating that the prescription was filled at the central fill pharmacy, in addition to the information required above.

These labeling requirements do not apply when a Schedule III, IV, or V controlled substance is prescribed for administration to an ultimate user who is institutionalized, provided that:

- not more than a 34-day supply or 100 dosage units, whichever is less, of the controlled substance listed in Schedule III, IV, or V is dispensed at one time.
- the controlled substance listed in Schedule III, IV, or V is not in the possession of the ultimate user prior to administration.
- the institution maintains appropriate safeguards and records the proper administration, control, dispensing, and storage of the Schedule III, IV, or V controlled substances.
- the system employed by the pharmacist in filling a prescription is adequate to identify the supplier, the product and the patient, and to include the directions for use and cautionary statements, if any, contained in the prescription or required by law.

Transfer of Prescription Information Between Pharmacies

Original prescription information for a Schedule III, IV or V controlled substance may be transferred on a one-time basis only for the purpose of refill dispensing.

Pharmacies electronically sharing a real-time online database may transfer up to the maximum refills permitted by law and the prescriber's authorization.

All transfers of Schedule III, IV or V controlled substance prescription information are subject to the following requirements:

- The transfer is communicated directly between two licensed pharmacists and the transferring pharmacist completes the following:
  - — Writes the word "VOID" on the face of the invalidated prescription. For electronic prescriptions, information that the prescription has been transferred must be added to the prescription record.
  - — Records on the reverse side of the invalidated prescription the name, address and DEA registration number of the pharmacy to which it was transferred and the name of the pharmacist receiving the prescription information. For electronic prescriptions, such information must be added to the prescription record.
  - — Records the date of the transfer and the name of the pharmacist transferring the information.
- For paper prescriptions and prescriptions received orally and reduced to writing by the pharmacist pursuant to the CSA, the pharmacist receiving the transferred prescription information must write the word "transfer" on the face of the transferred prescription and reduce to writing all information required by CSA to be on a prescription, including:
  - — Writing the word "TRANSFER" on the face of the transferred prescription.
  - — Entering all information required by the CSA on the prescription, including the:
    - ✧ date of issuance of original prescription.
    - ✧ original number of refills authorized on the original prescription.
    - ✧ date of original dispensing.
    - ✧ number of valid refills remaining.
    - ✧ date(s) and locations of previous refill(s).
    - ✧ pharmacy's name, address, DEA registration number

and prescription number from which the prescription information was transferred.

- ✧ name of pharmacist who transferred the prescription.
- ✧ pharmacy's name, address, DEA registration number and prescription number from which the prescription was originally filled.

- The original and transferred prescription(s) must be maintained for a period of two years from the date of last refill.

The pharmacist receiving a transferred electronic prescription must create an electronic record for the prescription that includes the receiving pharmacist's name and all of the information transferred with the prescription as described above.

Pharmacies electronically accessing the same prescription record must satisfy all the same information requirements as for the transfer of manual prescriptions.

The procedure allowing the transfer of prescription information for refill purposes is permissible only if allowable under existing state or other applicable law.

Dispensing Schedule V Controlled Substances Without a Prescription

A Schedule V controlled substance that is not a prescription drug pursuant to any federal, state or local law may be dispensed by a pharmacist without a prescription to a retail purchaser provided that:

- such dispensing is made only by a pharmacist, and not by a non-pharmacist employee even if under the supervision of a pharmacist (although after the pharmacist has fulfilled his/her professional and legal responsibilities, the actual cash, credit transaction, or delivery, may be completed by a non-pharmacist).

> **Note**
>
> Only a pharmacist may dispense an OTC Schedule V controlled substance, although a non-pharmacist may complete the sale.

- not more than
  - 240 mL (8 ounces) of any such controlled substance containing opium, or
  - 120 mL (4 fluid ounces) of any other such controlled substance, or
  - 48 dosage units of any such controlled substance containing opium, or
  - 24 dosage units of any other such controlled substance

  may be dispensed at retail to the same purchaser in any given 48-hour period.

> **Note**
>
> Therefore, a pharmacist who sells a codeine-containing cough preparation over-the-counter may not sell more than 4 fluid ounces to a given purchaser in any 48-hour period.

- the purchaser is at least 18 years of age.
- the pharmacist must require every purchaser of a controlled substance not known to him/her to furnish suitable identification (including proof of age where appropriate).
- a bound record book for dispensing controlled substances without a prescription must be maintained by the pharmacist. The

book must contain the

- — name and address of each purchaser.
- — name and quantity of controlled substance purchased.
- — date of each purchase.
- — name or initials of the pharmacist who dispensed the substance to the purchaser.

The record book must be maintained as other records described in the CSA for a period of at least two years.

Central fill pharmacies may not dispense controlled substances to a purchaser at retail.

Communicating prescription information between retail pharmacies and central fill pharmacies for initial and refill prescriptions of Schedule III, IV, or V controlled substances.

Prescriptions for controlled substances listed in Schedule III, IV or V may be transmitted electronically from a retail pharmacy to a central fill pharmacy including via facsimile. The retail pharmacy transmitting the prescription information must:

(1) Write the word "CENTRAL FILL" on the face of the original prescription and record the name, address, and DEA registration number of the central fill pharmacy to which the prescription has been transmitted and the name of the retail pharmacy pharmacist transmitting the prescription, and the date of transmittal;

(2) Ensure that all information required to be on a prescription as required by the CSA is transmitted to the central fill pharmacy (either on the face of the prescription or in the electronic transmission of information);

(3) Indicate in the information transmitted the number of refills already dispensed and the number of refills remaining;

(4) Maintain the original prescription for a period of two years from the date the prescription was last refilled;

(5) Keep a record of receipt of the filled prescription, including the date of receipt, the method of delivery (private, common or contract carrier) and the name of the retail pharmacy employee accepting delivery.

The central fill pharmacy receiving the transmitted prescription must:

(1) Keep a copy of the prescription (if sent via facsimile) or an electronic record of all the information transmitted by the retail pharmacy, including the name, address, and DEA registration number of the retail pharmacy transmitting the prescription;

(2) Keep a record of the date of receipt of the transmitted prescription, the name of the licensed pharmacist filling the prescription, and dates of filling or refilling of the prescription;

(3) Keep a record of the date the filled prescription was delivered to the retail pharmacy and the method of delivery (i.e. private, common or contract carrier).

Disposal of Controlled Substances

A pharmacy may transfer controlled substances to a DEA registered reverse distributor who handles the disposal of controlled substances. The pharmacy should contact the local DEA Diversion Field Office for an updated list of DEA registered reverse distributors. In no case should drugs be forwarded to the DEA unless the registrant has received prior approval from the DEA. The DEA procedures established for the disposal of controlled substances must not be construed as altering in any way the state laws or regulations for the disposal of controlled substances.

When a pharmacy transfers schedule II controlled substances to a reverse distributor for destruction, the reverse distributor must issue an official order form (DEA Form 222) or the electronic equivalent to the pharmacy. When schedules III-V controlled substances are transferred to a reverse distributor for destruction, the pharmacy must maintain a record of distribution that lists the drug name, dosage form, strength, quantity, and date transferred. The DEA registered reverse distributor who will destroy the controlled substances is responsible for submitting a DEA Form 41 to the DEA when the controlled substances have been destroyed. A DEA Form 41 should not be used to record the transfer of controlled substances between the pharmacy and the reverse distributor disposing of the drugs.

Note

Remember that many states have their own laws regarding the destruction of controlled substances. It is essential that you review the pertinent laws in your state to assure that these actions are performed correctly.

Transfer of Controlled Substances Between Pharmacies

A pharmacy practitioner who is registered to dispense controlled substances may distribute (without being registered to distribute) a quantity of such substance to another pharmacy practitioner for the purpose of general dispensing to his/her patients, provide that the practitioner to whom the controlled substance is to be distributed is registered under the Controlled Substances Act to dispense that controlled substance and that

- the distribution is recorded by the distributing practitioner and by the receiving practitioner;
- if the substance is listed in Schedule I or II, an order form (DEA Form 222) is used;
- the total number of dosage units of all controlled substances

distributed by the practitioner during each calendar year in which the practitioner is registered to dispense does not exceed five percent of the total number of dosage units of all controlled substances distributed and dispensed by the practitioner during the same calendar year;

- if, during any calendar year in which the pharmacy practitioner is registered to dispense, he/she has reason to believe that the total number of dosage units of all controlled substances which will be distributed by him/her will exceed five percent of the total number of dosage units of all controlled substances distributed and dispensed by him/her during that calendar year, the practitioner must obtain a registration to distribute controlled substances.

> **Note**
>
> In other words, a pharmacist may transfer up to 5% of the total dosage units of controlled substances dispensed in a given calendar year by the pharmacy without getting a wholesaler's permit. DEA Form 222 must also be used in transferring Schedule I and/or II controlled substances to another pharmacy.

If a pharmacy goes out of business or is acquired by a new pharmacy, it may transfer the controlled substances to another pharmacy, supplier, manufacturer or distributor registered to dispose of controlled substances.

To transfer Schedule II substances, the receiving registrant must issue an Official Order Form (DEA Form 222) to the registrant transferring the drugs.

The transfer of Schedule III-V controlled substances must be documented in writing to show the drug name, dosage form, strength, quantity and date transferred. The document must include the names, addresses and DEA registration numbers of the parties involved in the transfer of the controlled substances.

If a pharmacy going out of business wishes to transfer its controlled substances to another pharmacy, the pharmacy must, on the day the controlled substances are transferred, take a complete inventory, which documents the drugs' name, dosage form, strength, quantity, and date transferred. In addition, a DEA Form 222 must be prepared to document the transfer of Schedule II controlled substances. This inventory will serve as the final inventory for the registrant going out of business and transferring the controlled substances. It will also serve as the initial inventory for the registrant acquiring the controlled substances. A copy of the inventory must be included in the records of each person. It is not necessary to send a copy of the inventory to the DEA. The person acquiring the controlled substances must maintain all records involved in the transfer of the controlled substances for at least two years.

Controlled Substance Records

Prescribers

Prescribers are required to keep records of controlled substances in schedules II, III, IV, and V that are dispensed, other than by prescribing or administering, in their practice. Such practitioners are NOT required to keep records of controlled substances in schedules II, III, IV, and V which are prescribed in the lawful course of their practice, unless such substances are prescribed as part of a maintenance or detoxification treatment of an individual.

Prescribers are not required to keep records of controlled substances listed in Schedules II, III, IV and V that are administered in their practice unless the prescriber regularly engages in the dispensing or administering of controlled substances and charges patients, either separately or together, with charges for other professional services, for substances so dispensed or administered.

Records must be kept for controlled substances administered in the course of maintenance or detoxification treatment of an individual.

Mid-level Practitioners

Each registered mid-level practitioner must maintain, in a readily retrievable manner, those documents required by the state in which he/she practices, which describe the conditions and extent of his/her authorization to dispense controlled substances. The practitioner must make such documents available for inspection and copying by authorized employees of the DEA. Examples of such documentation include protocols, practice guidelines or practice agreements.

Pharmacists

Each registered pharmacy must maintain the following inventories and records of controlled substances:

- Inventories and records of all controlled substances listed in Schedules I and II must be maintained separately from all other records of the pharmacy, and prescriptions for such substances must be maintained in a separate prescription file.
- Inventories and records of controlled substances listed in Schedules III, IV, and V must be maintained either separately from all other records of the pharmacy or in such form that the information required is readily retrievable from ordinary business records of the pharmacy. Prescriptions for such substances must be maintained either in a separate prescription file for controlled substances listed in Schedules III, IV, and V only or in such form that they are readily retrievable from the other prescription records of the pharmacy.
- Prescriptions will be deemed readily retrievable if, at the time they are initially filed, the face of the prescription is stamped in red ink in the lower right corner with the letter "C" no less than one inch high and filed either in the prescription file for controlled substances listed in Schedules I and II or in the customary consecutively numbered prescription file for non-controlled substances.

- If a pharmacy employs a computer system or other electronic record-keeping system for prescriptions that permits identification by prescription number and retrieval of original documents by prescriber's name, patient's name, drug dispensed, and date filled, then the requirement to mark the hard copy prescription with a red "C" is waived.

> ***Note***
>
> Schedule III, IV, or V prescriptions need NOT be stamped with the red letter "C" if a computer record of these prescriptions is maintained.

Other Entities

Each registered manufacturer, distributor, importer, exporter, narcotic treatment program and compounder for a narcotic treatment program must maintain the following inventories and records of controlled substances:

- Inventories and records of controlled substances listed in Schedules I and II must be maintained separately from all of the records of the Registrant; and
- Inventories and records of controlled substances listed in Schedules III, IV, and V must be maintained either separately from all other records of the registrant or in such form that the information required is readily retrievable from the ordinary business records of the registrant.

Inventory Requirements

Every required inventory and other records must be kept by the registrant and be available, for at least 2 years from the date of such inventory or records, for inspection and copying by authorized employees of the DEA.

Records and inventories of Schedule II controlled substances must be maintained separately from all other records of the registrant. All records and inventories of Schedule III, IV and V controlled substances must be maintained either separately from all other records or in such a form that the information required is readily retrievable from the ordinary business records.

Financial and shipping records (such as invoices and packing slips) may be kept at a central location (e.g. at the main office of a chain pharmacy), rather than at the registered location, if the registrant has notified the DEA of his/her intention to keep central records.

Each controlled substance inventory must contain a complete and accurate record of all controlled substances on hand on the date the inventory is taken, and must be maintained in written, typewritten, or printed form at the registered location. An inventory taken by use of an oral recording device must be promptly transcribed.

Controlled substances must be inventoried if they are in the possession of, or under the control of the registrant. These include substances

- returned by a customer.
- ordered by a customer but not yet invoiced.
- stored in a warehouse on behalf of the registrant.
- in the possession of employees of the registrant and intended for distribution as complimentary samples.

A separate inventory must be made for each registered location and each independent activity registered. In the event controlled substances in the possession or under the control of the registrant are stored at a location for which he/she is not registered, the substances must be included in the inventory of the registered location to which they are subject to control or to which the person possessing the substance is responsible.

The inventory may be taken either as of opening of business or as of the close of business on the inventory date and this must be indicated on the inventory.

Every registrant is required to take an inventory of all stocks of controlled substances on hand on the date he/she first engages in the manufacture, distribution, or dispensing of controlled substances. In the event a person commences business with no controlled substances on hand, he/she must record this fact as the initial inventory.

After the initial inventory is taken, the registrant must take a new inventory of all stocks of controlled substances on hand at least every two years. The biennial inventory may be taken on any date that is within two years of the previous biennial inventory date. The person conducting the inventory should sign the inventory.

Note

A controlled substance inventory must be taken at least once every two years.

When the status of a non-controlled substance is changed to that of a controlled substance or when a drug is moved from one controlled substance schedule to another, each registrant who possesses that substance must take an inventory of all stocks of the substance on hand on the date the change is made. Thereafter, the substance must be included in each inventory made by the registrant.

When conducting a controlled substance inventory, the registrant must make an exact count of substances in sealed, unopened containers. For opened containers the following should be performed:

- If the substance is listed in Schedule I or II, make an exact count or measure of the contents.
- If the substance is listed in Schedule III, IV or V, make an estimated count or measure of the contents, unless the container

holds more than 1,000 tablets or capsules in which case an exact count of the contents must be made.

Every registrant must maintain, on a current basis, a complete and accurate record of each controlled substance manufactured, imported, received, sold, delivered, exported, or otherwise disposed of. The records must be maintained in a dispensing log at the registered site. No registrant is required to maintain a perpetual inventory.

Each person registered or authorized to maintain and/or detoxify users of controlled substance, as part of a narcotic treatment program, must maintain records with the following information for each narcotic controlled substance:

- Name of substance
- Strength of substance
- Dosage form
- Date dispensed
- Adequate identification of patient (consumer)
- Amount consumed
- Amount and dosage form taken home by patient
- Dispenser's initials

All sites that compound a bulk narcotic solution from bulk narcotic powder into a liquid for on-site use must keep a separate batch record of the compounding.

Records of identity, diagnosis, prognosis, or treatment of any patients, which are maintained in connection with the operation of a narcotic treatment program, must be confidential.

Extensive record keeping is required of individuals authorized to compound narcotic drugs for off-site use in a narcotic treatment program.

Verification of DEA Numbers

Knowing how a DEA registration number is constructed can be

a useful tool for recognizing a forged prescription. Prior to October 1, 1985, DEA Registration numbers for physicians, dentists, veterinarians and other practitioners started with the letter A. Registration numbers issued to practitioners after that date begin with the letter B. As the registration numbers beginning with the letter B are exhausted, the DEA will issue practitioner registration numbers beginning with the letter F. Registration numbers issued to mid-level practitioners begin with the letter M. The first letter of the registrant's last name or business name follows the first letter of the registration number. (e.g., J for Jones), and then a computer generated sequence of seven numbers (e.g. MJ3614511).

A pharmacist may verify a prescriber's DEA number by performing the following calculation:

Assuming that the DEA number to verify is BR2398328

- Add the 1st, 3rd, and 5th digits of the number

  2 + 9 + 3 = 14

- Add the 2nd, 4th, and 6th digits of the number and multiply this sum by 2.

  3 +8 + 2 = 13 13 x 2 = 26

- Add the results of the first two calculations

  14 + 26 = 40

The last digit of this final sum (in this case, "0") should be the same as the last digit (i.e. the 7th and final digit) of the DEA number being tested. Since the last digit of the DEA number provided is "8", it is not a valid DEA number. The final number should be "0" to make it a valid number.

Prescribing by Hospital Employees

An individual practitioner (e.g., intern, resident, staff physician, mid-level practitioner) who is an agent or employee of a hospital or other institution may, when acting in the usual course of business or employment, administer, dispense or prescribe controlled substances under the registration of the hospital or other institution in which the practitioner is employed, provided that:

- the dispensing, administering, or prescribing is in the usual course of the practitioner's professional practice;
- the practitioner is authorized to do so by the state in which he or she is practicing;
- the hospital or institution has verified that the practitioner is permitted to dispense, administer or prescribe controlled substances within the state;
- the practitioner acts only within the scope of their employment in the hospital or institution;
- the hospital or institution authorizes the practitioner to dispense or prescribe under its registration and assigns a specific internal code number for each practitioner so authorized (See example of a specific internal code number below);

AB1234567-012

Hospital DEA Registration Number	Physician's Hospital Code Number

The hospital or other institution should keep a current list of internal codes and the corresponding individual practitioners. This list must be available at all times to other registrants and law enforcement agencies upon request for the purpose of verifying the authority of the prescribing individual practitioner. Pharmacists should contact the hospital or other institution for verification if they have any doubts in dispensing such a prescription.

Mid-level Practitioners (MLP)

Mid-level practitioners (MLP) are registered and authorized by the DEA and the state in which they practice to dispense, administer and prescribe controlled substances in the course of their professional practice. Examples of MLPs include, but are not limited to, health care providers such as nurse practitioners, nurse midwives, nurse anesthetists, clinical nurse specialists, physician assistants, optometrists, ambulance services, animal shelters, veterinarian euthanasia technicians, nursing homes and homeopathic physicians.

MLPs may receive an individual DEA registration granting controlled substance privileges. However, such a registration is contingent upon authority granted by the state in which they are licensed. The DEA registers MLPs whose states clearly authorize them to prescribe, dispense, and administer controlled substances in one or more schedules. The fact that a MLP has been issued a valid DEA registration number (beginning with the letter M) will be evidence that the practitioner is authorized to prescribe, dispense and/or administer at least some controlled substances. However, it will still be incumbent upon the pharmacist who fills the prescription to ensure that the MLP is prescribing within the parameters established by the state in which the practitioner practices.

MLP authority to prescribe controlled substances varies greatly by state. Check with your state licensing or controlled substances authority to determine which MLP disciplines are authorized to prescribe controlled substances in your state.

Storage of Controlled Substances

Practitioners and non-practitioners authorized to conduct research or chemical analysis must store controlled substances listed in Schedules II, III, IV, and V in a securely locked, substantially constructed cabinet. However, pharmacies and institutional practitioners may store controlled substances by

- keeping them in a locked secure cabinet.
- dispersing them throughout the stock of non-controlled substances in such a manner as to obstruct the theft or diversion.

An electronic alarm system is also recommended.

Carfentanil, etorphine hydrochloride and diprenorphine must be stored in a safe or steel cabinet equivalent to a U.S. Government Class V security container.

Pharmacy Employment Practices

A pharmacy registrant (i.e., the registrant or corporation that owns the pharmacy) must not employ in a position, which allows access to controlled substances, anyone who has been convicted of a felony relating to controlled substances, or who, at any time, has had an application for DEA registration denied, revoked, or surrendered for cause. "For cause" means surrendering a registration in lieu of, or as a consequence of, any federal or state administrative, civil or criminal action resulting from an investigation of the individual's handling of controlled substances.

Pharmacies desiring to employ an individual who meets this definition may request an exception to this requirement from the DEA. The employer must have a waiver approved before hiring the applicant. A waiver request should be sent to DEA Headquarters, Office of Diversion Control, Washington, D.C. 20537.

A pharmacy registrant who applies for such a waiver should understand that the following factors will be considered:

- A detailed description of the nature and extent of the applicant's past controlled substances violations
- Activities of the applicant since the violation
- Current status of the applicant's state licensure
- Extent of the applicant's proposed access to controlled substances
- Registrant's proposed physical and professional safeguards to prevent diversion by the applicant, if employed

- Status of employing registrant regarding handling of controlled substances
- Other pertinent information uncovered by DEA in its investigation of the applicant's or registrant's handling of controlled substances

Such a waiver should not be considered unless there are valid reasons to believe that diversion is unlikely to occur.

Theft of Controlled Substances

Immediately upon discovery of a theft or significant loss of controlled substances, a pharmacy must contact the nearest DEA Diversion Field Office by telephone, facsimile or by a brief written message explaining the circumstances. A pharmacy should also notify the local police as may be required by state law. If there is a question as to whether a theft has occurred or a loss is significant, a registrant should err on the side of caution and report it to DEA.

The DEA must be notified directly. Reporting the theft or significant loss in any other manner does not satisfy this requirement. For example, a corporation, which owns or operates multiple registered sites and wishes to channel all notifications through corporate management or any other internal department responsible for security, must still provide notice directly to DEA "upon discovery" and keep a copy for its records.

A pharmacy must also complete a DEA Form 106 (Report of Theft or Loss of Controlled Substances). The DEA Form 106 will formally document the actual circumstances of the theft or significant loss and the quantities of controlled substances involved, once this information has been determined conclusively. The pharmacy should send the original DEA Form 106 and a copy to the DEA Diversion Field Office and keep a copy for its records.

When all or part of a shipment disappears, or never reaches its intended destination, the supplier is responsible for reporting the in-transit loss of controlled substances to DEA. A pharmacy is responsible for reporting any loss of controlled substances after a pharmacist has signed for or taken custody of a shipment. If it's discovered, after the pharmacist has taken custody of a shipment, that an in-transit loss or theft has occurred, the pharmacist must submit a DEA Form 106.

If, after an investigation of the circumstances surrounding an alleged theft or significant loss, it is determined that no such theft or significant loss occurred, no DEA Form 106 need be filed. However, the registrant should notify DEA in writing of this fact in order to resolve the initial report and explain why no DEA Form 106 was filed regarding the incident.

Breakage, damage or spillage does not constitute a "loss of controlled substances". In such situations, any recoverable controlled substances must be disposed of according to DEA requirements, and a DEA Form 41 should be filed.

Federal Investigation of Pharmaceutical Theft or Robbery

The Controlled Substances Registrant Protection Act of 1984 (CSRPA) provides for the federal investigation of pharmaceutical thefts and robberies if any of the following conditions are met:

- Replacement cost of the controlled substances taken is $500 or more.
- A registrant or other person is killed or suffers "significant" bodily injury during the commission of the robbery or theft of a controlled substance.
- Interstate or foreign commerce is involved in planning or executing the crime.

Required Records

A registrant must maintain the following records:

- Official order forms (DEA Form 222).

- Power of Attorney authorization to sign order forms.
- Receipts and invoices for Schedule III, IV, and V controlled substances.
- All inventory records of controlled substances, including the initial and biennial inventories.
- Records of controlled substances distributed or dispensed (i.e., prescriptions).
- Report of Theft or Loss (DEA Form 106).
- Inventory of Drugs Surrendered for Disposal (DEA Form 41).
- Records of transfers of controlled substances between pharmacies.
- DEA registration certificate.

> **Study Hint**
>
> This list provides a great review of documents that you must be familiar with. If you still don't understand the use of each of these records, review previous sections.

Storing Prescription Information

Pharmacies have three options for filing prescription records under the Code of Federal Regulations. If there is a conflict between federal and state requirements for filing prescriptions, DEA recognizes that the pharmacy must choose a filing system that would comply with both federal and state law.

All prescription records must be readily retrievable for DEA inspection. Controlled substance prescriptions must be filed in one of the following three ways:

Option 1 (Three separate files)

- A file for Schedule II drugs dispensed.
- A file for Schedule III, IV and V drugs dispensed.
- A file for prescription orders for all noncontrolled drugs dispensed.

Option 2 (Two separate files)

- A file for all Schedule II drugs dispensed.
- A file for all other drugs dispensed (non-controlled and those in Schedule III, IV and V). If this method is used, a prescription for a Schedule III, IV and V drug must be made readily identifiable and retrievable by use of a red "C" stamp not less than one inch high. (See Note below).

Option 3 (Two separate files)

- A file for all Schedules II-V controlled substances. If this method is used, a prescription for a Schedule III, IV and V drug must be made readily retrievable by use of a red "C" stamp not less than one inch high. (See Note below).
- A file for prescription orders for all noncontrolled drugs dispensed.

Note

If a pharmacy has an electronic recordkeeping system for prescriptions, which permits identification by prescription number and retrieval of original documents by prescriber's name, patient's name, drug dispensed and date filled, then the requirements to mark the hard copy prescription with a red "C" is waived.

A pharmacy is permitted to use a data processing system as an alternative to the manual method for the storage and retrieval of prescription order refill information for Schedules III, IV and V controlled substances. The computer system must provide online retrieval of original prescription information for those prescriptions, which are currently authorized for refill. The information must include, but is not limited to, the original prescription number, date of issuance, full name and address of the patient, the prescriber's name, address, and DEA registration number; the name, strength, dosage form and quantity of the controlled substance prescribed; and the total number of refills authorized by the prescriber. In addition, the computer system must provide online retrieval of the current refill history for Schedule III, IV, or V controlled substance prescriptions. This information must include, but is not limited to the:

- name of the controlled substance.
- date of refill.
- quantity dispensed.
- dispensing pharmacist's identification code, or name/initials for each refill.
- total number of refills dispensed to date for that prescription.

The pharmacist must verify and document that the refill data entered into the system is correct. All computer generated prescription or refill documentation must be stored in a separate file at the pharmacy and be maintained for a two-year period from the dispensing date.

The pharmacy's computer system must comply with the following guidelines:

- If the system provides a hard copy printout of each day's controlled substance prescription refills, each pharmacist who refilled those prescriptions must verify their accuracy by signing and dating the printout, as they would sign a check or legal document.

- This printout must be provided to each pharmacy, which uses the computer system within 72 hours of the date on which the refill was dispensed. The printout must be verified and signed by each pharmacist who dispensed the refills in the pharmacy.
- In lieu of such a printout, the pharmacy must maintain a bound log book, or separate file in which each pharmacist involved in the day's dispensing signs a statement verifying that the refill information entered into the computer that day has been carefully reviewed by him/her and is correct.
- A pharmacy computer system must have the capability of printing out any refill data, which the pharmacy must maintain under the Controlled Substances Act. For example, this would include a refill-by-refill audit trail for any specified strength and dosage form of any controlled substance, by either brand or generic name or both, dispensed by the pharmacy. Such a printout must include the:
  - — prescribing practitioner's name.
  - — patient's name and address.
  - — quantity dispensed on each refill.
  - — dispensing date for each refill.
  - — name or identification code of the dispensing pharmacist.
  - — original prescription number.

In any computerized system employed by a user pharmacy, the central recordkeeping location must be capable of providing a printout to a requesting pharmacy of the above information within 48 hours.

In case a pharmacy's computer system experiences downtime, the pharmacy must have a back-up procedure to document in writing refills of Schedule III, IV and V substances. This procedure must ensure that refills are authorized by the original prescription, that the maximum number of refills has not been exceeded, and that all required data is retained for online entry as soon as possible.

A pharmacy may use only one of the two systems described (i.e., manual or computer).

Exportation of Controlled Substances

The Controlled Substances Act of 1970 (CSA) placed severe restrictions on the exportation of controlled substances from the US to other countries and limited their exportation only to countries that were part of international controlled substance agreements. Furthermore, controlled substances could only be exported to countries where the drugs were to be directly consumed, thereby preventing export of these drugs to other countries. This jeopardized the ability of American pharmaceutical manufacturers to have drug warehouses and distribution facilities in other countries.

In 2005 the Controlled Substances Export Reform Act was passed. This law authorizes the Attorney General (or his designee, the DEA) to permit re-export of controlled substances in categories I-IV to other countries as long as they are being shipped to DEA permit or license holders in those countries and as long as DEA is notified of the re-export within 30 days.

Methamphetamine Anti-Proliferation

A number of pieces of federal legislation have been directed at reducing the production and distribution of methamphetamine in the US. The Methamphetamine Anti-Proliferation Act (MAPA) of 2000 addresses issues ranging from the diversion of drug products containing pseudoephedrine (PSE) and phenylpropanolamine (PPA) from retail and mail order sources to the illicit production of methamphetamine.

In 2006, President George W. Bush signed into law the USA Patriot Act, Title VII, which includes the Combat Methamphetamine Epidemic Act (CMEA) of 2005. This federal law applies to all cough and cold products (including combination products) that contain the methamphetamine precursor chemicals ephedrine, pseudoephedrine, or phenylpropanolamine. All PSE products, including liquids, gelcaps, and pediatrics, are subject to the law. Products reformulated so that they no longer contain these precursors may be sold without regard to the new statutory provisions. The following are the other critical elements of this law:

1. Retail sales may not exceed 3.6 grams PSE per day per purchaser, regardless of the number of transactions.
2. Individuals are prohibited from purchasing more than 9 grams of PSE per 30-day period.
3. All non-liquid forms (including gelcaps) of PSE products must be sold in blister packs with no more than two dosages or in unit-dose packets or pouches.
4. Mail-order companies may not sell more than 7.5 grams of PSE to a customer within a 30-day period.
5. All PSE products must be placed behind a counter (any counter, not necessarily the pharmacy counter) that is not accessible to purchasing consumers, or in a locked display case that is located on the selling floor. Retailers must give the product directly to the purchaser.
6. A retailer without a pharmacy may still sell the combination PSE products from behind a counter or locked display case.
7. Retailers must maintain a logbook of information on transactions involving PSE products. The logbook may be maintained in either written or electronic form.
8. The purchaser must enter onto the log their signature, their name and address, and the date and time of the sale. The retailer must check the entered information against a photo ID issued by either a state or the federal government, or other appropriate ID, and enter the name of the product sold and quantity sold.
9. Logbooks must provide notice to purchasers that entering false statements or misrepresentations in the logbook may subject them to criminal penalties.

10. Logbook requirements do not apply to purchases of single sales packages that contain no more than 60 mg of PSE. Each entry must be maintained for two years from the date of entry.
11. Retailers must train applicable sales personnel to ensure that they understand the requirements of PSE product sales and submit self-certifications to the attorney general in this regard.

> **Note**
>
> 1. All of these requirements deal with nonprescription sales of these drugs. This includes gelcaps, liquids and pediatric dosage forms.
> 2. All non-liquid dosage forms of these products must be packaged in blister or unit-dose packaging with not more than two doses per blister pack.
> 3. Nonprescription phenylpropanolamine (PPA) products are no longer available in the United States or Canada because the use of PPA has been associated with elevated risk of hemorrhagic stroke in women and possibly in men.

Marijuana Prescribing and Dispensing

In 1996, California voters passed Proposition 215, making California the first in the union to allow for the medical use of marijuana. Since then, at least 24 more states, including the District of Columbia and Guam have enacted similar laws.

A number of states allow use of low levels of tetrahydrocannabinol (THC), high levels of cannabidiol (CBD) products. This reflects the fact that THC is believed to be the principal psychoactive constituent of cannabis while CBD is considered to have a broad scope of potential medical applications.

The therapeutic value of cannabinoid drugs, primarily THC, has been claimed to include pain relief, control of nausea and vomiting, and appetite stimulation. Smoked marijuana is considered to be a crude THC delivery system and may deliver harmful substances. The psychological effects of cannabinoids, such as anxiety reduction, sedation, and euphoria may potentially be undesirable for certain patients and beneficial for others. There have been some studies that indicated that marijuana may have possible uses in relieving some of the symptoms of HIV/AIDS, cancer, glaucoma, and multiple sclerosis.

As of the middle of 2016, the federal government classified marijuana as a Schedule I substance under the Controlled Substances Act, thereby not acknowledging the medicinal use of this drug. There is a growing likelihood that this will be changed to a Schedule II status in the immediate future. This would legalize the use of marijuana for medical uses and permit fewer conflicts between the federal and state governments.

Currently, most states with medical marijuana laws generally have some form of patient registry, which may provide some protection against arrest for possession up to a certain amount of marijuana for personal medicinal use.

If the federal government recognizes the medical benefits of marijuana use and reclassifies the drug to Schedule II, it is likely that there will be more consistency throughout the US with regard to prescribing, dispensing, and registration of approved patients.

Sample Questions

1. A suppository dosage form of secobarbital is likely to be classified in which of the following controlled substance schedules?

   (A) I (B) II (C) III (D) IV (E) V

2. DEA Form 222 must be used when which of the following classes of controlled substances are purchased?

I. Schedule I

II. Schedule II

III. Schedule III

(A) I only (B) III only (C) I & II only
(D) II & III only (E) I, II & III

3. Which of the following digits would make the following an authentic DEA number? BC445987__

(A) 6 (B) 7 (C) 8 (D) 9 (E) 0

4. A prescriber may authorize a maximum of how many refills on a prescription for Percodan tablets?

(A) 0 (B) 1 (C) 2 (D) 5 (E) 10

5. What percentage of the controlled substance doses dispensed each year may be transferred to another pharmacy without requiring registration as a wholesaler?

(A) 0 (B) 5 (C) 7 (D) 10 (E) 20

6. A partial filling of a Schedule II prescription is permissible under which of the following circumstances?

I. The patient is over 65 and only wants half the number of doses prescribed by the physician because he cannot afford the full amount.

II. The prescriber indicates that she would like the patient to get half the prescription today and the rest in a week if the medication agrees with him.

III. The pharmacist is out of stock and will provide the balance of the prescription to the patient in two days.

(A) I only (B) III only (C) I & II only
(D) II & III only (E) I, II & III

7. A product that contains not more than 200 mg of codeine per 100 mL of product is classified in controlled substance category:

(A) noncontrolled
(B) Schedule II
(C) Schedule III
(D) Schedule IV
(E) Schedule V

8. When using a DEA Form 222, the center portion of the 3-part form ultimately ends up with the

(A) purchaser
(B) state board of pharmacy
(C) supplier
(D) regional poison control center
(E) DEA

9. Which of the following hospital employees may be permitted to prescribe controlled substances even though they do not have a DEA registration number?

I. Medical Interns
II. Medical Residents
III. Mid-level practitioners

(A) I only
(B) III only
(C) I & II only
(D) II & III only
(E) I, II & III

10. Controlled substances may be stored in a pharmacy

I. on a controlled substance shelf in the pharmacy department.
II. dispersed through the pharmacy department with non-controlled drug products.
III. in a securely locked cabinet

(A) I only
(B) III only
(C) I & II only
(D) II & III only
(E) I, II & III

11. Nonprescription products containing which of the following drugs must not be directly accessible to the consumer?

I. phenylpropanolamine

II. pseudoephedrine

III. dextromethorphan

(A) I only (B) III only (C) I & II only

(D) II & III only (E) I, II & III

12. Which one of the following acronyms represent a method acceptable by the DSA for ordering Schedule II substances?

(A) DSA-II (B) CSOS (C) SIIO

(D) NDC (E) EOB

Answers:

(1) C (2) C (3) B (4) A (5) B (6) B
(7) E (8) E (9) E (10) D (11) C (12) B

Section I

Treatment of Narcotic Dependence

The use of methadone as a way to wean narcotic-dependent individuals from opiates began with the passage of the Comprehensive Drug Abuse Prevention and Control Act of 1970. This approach to treatment has been very controversial because methadone itself is a controlled substance capable of being abused and has at times been diverted into illicit channels. The Narcotic Addict Treatment Act (NATA) of 1974 provided for more stringent controls of methadone use and restricts its dispensing to practitioners who are registered with DEA and in compliance with the Drug Abuse Prevention and Control Act.

The Drug Addiction Treatment Act of 2000 (DATA 2000) provides a waiver from the NATA requirements and permits qualified office-based physicians to prescribe and pharmacists to dispense schedule III, IV, or V narcotic drugs, or combinations of such drugs, approved by the FDA for the treatment of opioid addiction. In order to qualify for a waiver under DATA 2000, physicians must hold a current state medical license, a valid DEA registration number, and must meet a variety of special conditions.

In addition, physicians must attest that they have the capacity to refer addiction treatment patients for appropriate counseling and other non-pharmacological therapies, and that they will not have more than 30 patients on such addiction treatment at any one time.

Use of Buprenorphine Products

In October 2002 The FDA approved the use of Subutex® (buprenorphine HCl) and Suboxone® (buprenorphine HCl + naloxone) sublingual tablets for the treatment of opioid dependence.

Since both of these products contain buprenorphine HCl, a Schedule III drug, qualified office-based practitioners may prescribe it under the DATA 2000 regulations. It is recommended that Subutex® be given during the first few days of treatment, while Suboxone® be used during the maintenance phase of treatment.

Required Services for Opioid Treatment Programs (OTPs)

OTPs must provide adequate medical, counseling, vocational, educational, and other assessment and treatment services. These services must be available at the primary facility, except where the program sponsor has entered into a formal, documented agreement with a private or public agency, organization, practitioner, or institution to provide these services to patients enrolled in the OTP. The program sponsor, in any event, must be able to document that these services are fully and reason-ably available to patients.

OTPs must use only those opioid agonist treatment medications that are approved by the Food and Drug Administration for use in the treatment of opioid addiction. In addition, OTPs who are fully compliant with the protocol of an investigational use of a drug and other conditions set forth in the application may administer a drug that has been authorized by the Food and Drug Administration under an investigational new drug application for investigational use in the treatment of opioid addiction. Currently, the Food and Drug Administration has approved the following agents for use in the treatment of opioid addiction:

- **Methadone** is a slow-acting, opioid agonist. It is taken orally, so that it reaches the brain slowly, dampening the "high" that occurs with other routes of administration while preventing withdrawal symptoms. Methadone has been in use since the 1960s to treat heroin addiction and is still an excellent treatment option, particularly for patients that do not respond well to other medications. It is, however, only available through approved outpatient treatment programs, where it is dispensed to patients on a daily basis.

- **Buprenorphine HCl** (Subutex), is a partial opioid agonist. Subutex relieves drug cravings without producing the "high" or dangerous side effects of other opioids. Suboxone, which is taken orally, combines buprenorphine with naloxone (an opioid antagonist) to ward off attempts to get high by injecting the medication. If an addicted patient were to inject Suboxone, the naloxone would induce withdrawal symptoms, which are averted when taken orally as prescribed. The FDA approved buprenorphine in 2002, making it the first medication eligible to be prescribed by certified physicians through the Drug Addiction Treatment Act. This approval eliminates the need to visit specialized treatment clinics, expanding treatment access.
- **Naltrexone** (Depade, Revia) an opioid antagonist. It is not addictive or sedating and does not result in physical dependence; however, poor patient compliance has limited its effectiveness. Recently an long acting injectable formulation of naltrexone called Vivitrol received FDA approval for treating opioid addiction. Given as a monthly injection, Vivitrol may improve compliance by eliminating the need for daily dosing. To avoid withdrawal symptoms, Vivitrol should be used only after a patient has undergone detoxification. Vivitrol provides an effective alternative for individuals who are unable to or choose not to engage in agonist-assisted treatment.

OTPs must maintain current procedures that are adequate to ensure that the following dosage form and initial dosing requirements are met:

- Methadone must be administered or dispensed only in oral form and must be formulated in such a way as to reduce its potential for parenteral abuse. Practitioners may not prescribe these agents for treatment of drug dependence.
- For each new patient enrolled in a program, the initial dose of methadone must not exceed 30 milligrams and the total dose for the first day must not exceed 40 milligrams, unless the pro-

gram physician documents in the patient's record that 40 milligrams did not suppress opiate abstinence symptoms.

- A program physician familiar with the most up-to-date product labeling must make dosing and administration decisions in the use of these drugs. These procedures must ensure that any significant deviations from the approved labeling, including deviations with regard to dose, frequency, or the conditions of use described in the approved labeling, are specifically documented in the patient's record.

Prevention of Drug Diversion

To limit the potential for diversion of opioid agonist treatment medications to the illicit market, opioid agonist treatment medications dispensed to patients for unsupervised use are be subject to the following requirements:

- Any patient in a comprehensive maintenance treatment program may receive a single take-home dose for a day that the clinic is closed for business, including Sundays and state and federal holidays.
- Treatment program decisions for dispensing opioid treatment medications to patients for unsupervised use must be determined by the Medical Director. In determining which patients may be permitted unsupervised use, the Medical Director must consider the following take-home criteria in determining whether a patient is responsible in handling opioid drugs for unsupervised use.
  - — Absence of recent abuse of drugs (opioid or non-narcotic), including alcohol;
  - — Regularity of clinic attendance;
  - — Absence of serious behavioral problems at the clinic;
  - — Absence of known recent criminal activity, e.g., drug dealing;

— Stability of the patient's home environment and social relationships;

— Length of time in comprehensive maintenance treatment;

— Assurance that take-home medication can be safely stored within the patient's home; and

— Whether the rehabilitative benefit the patient derived from decreasing the frequency of clinic attendance outweighs the potential risks of diversion.

If it is determined that a patient is responsible in handling opioid drugs, the following restrictions apply:

- During the first 90 days of treatment, the take-home supply is limited to a single dose each week and the patient shall ingest all other doses under appropriate supervision.
- In the second 90 days of treatment, the take-home supply is two doses per week.
- In the third 90 days of treatment, the take-home supply is three doses per week.
- In the remaining months of the first year, a patient may be given a maximum 6-day supply of take-home medication.
- After one year of continuous treatment, a patient may be given a maximum 2-week supply of take-home medication.
- After two years of continuous treatment, a patient may be given a maximum one-month supply of take-home medication, but must make monthly visits.

No medications may be dispensed to patients in short-term detoxification treatment or interim maintenance treatment for unsupervised or take-home use.

OTPs must maintain current procedures adequate to identify the theft or diversion of take-home medications, including labeling containers with the OTP's name, address, and telephone number. Programs also must ensure that take-home supplies are packaged in a manner that is designed to reduce the risk of accidental ingestion, including the use of child-resistant containers.

Naloxone For Treatment of Opium and Opioid Overdose

Unintentional drug overdose of opium or opioids is a leading cause of preventable death in the United States. The administration of naloxone hydrochloride can rapidly and relatively safely reverse the effects of an opium or opioid overdose and prevent these unintentional deaths.

Naloxone can be administered by IM injection, intranasally, or by use of a ready-to-use auto injector (e.g. Evzio Auto-Injector).

Naloxone is classified by the US Food and Drug Administration as a prescription drug. Presumably, these federal laws determine how the drug is to be administered and by whom.

However, many states have passed laws that provide legal immunities for health care professionals that prescribe naloxone or lay people who may administer the drug to friends or family who may be at risk of a drug overdose. This creates legal problems since the prescription is provided to an individual who will be administering the naloxone product to a third party.

Recently, CVS has instituted in over 15 states the distribution of naloxone products without the need of a prescription . This program has been accomplished by the use of a physician-approved protocol as well as training of the pharmacists involved.

Section J

Nonprescription Drugs

General Labeling Requirements

Over-the-counter (OTC) or nonprescription status is granted to drugs and drug products that have been shown to be safe for use without a physician's supervision, are for conditions suitable for self-diagnosis, and have adequate written directions for self-use. Of major importance with OTC products is appropriate labeling. The FDA has, over the past decade, focused considerable attention on the development of legislation that would improve the safety and efficacy of OTC products.

The FDA requires that all nonprescription, over-the-counter (OTC) medicine labels have detailed usage and warning information, in a "Drug Facts" section, so consumers can properly choose and use the products. Below is an example of what elements an OTC "Drug Facts" section must have, in the order in which the information must appear on the label :

(1) **Active Ingredient** - Indicates the active therapeutic substance in the product as well as the amount of active ingredient per unit (i.e.. per capsule, per teaspoonful, etc.)

(2) **Uses** - Symptoms or diseases the product will treat or prevent.

(3) **Warnings**. May include

- when not to use the product;
- conditions that may require advice from a doctor before taking the product;
- possible interactions or side effects;
- when to stop taking the product and when to contact a doctor;

- The statement "If you are pregnant or breast feeding, seek guidance from a health care professional";
- The statement "Keep product out of children's reach".

(4) **Inactive Ingredients** - Lists substances such as colors or flavors.

(5) **Purpose** - Indicates the product's action or category (e.g. antihistamine, antacid, cough suppressant, etc.)

(6) **Directions** - Lists
- Specific age categories that may use the product
- How much to take
- How, how often, and how long to take.

(7) **Other Information** - May include
- How to store the product properly
- Required information about certain ingredients (such as the amount of calcium, potassium, or sodium the product contains).

If any of the above information is missing, the nonprescription product is considered misbranded.

In addition, the OTC label will generally have the following additional information:

- Expiration date, when applicable
- Lot or batch code (manufacturer information to help identify the product).
- Name and address of manufacturer, packer, or distributor.
- Net quantity of contents (how much of the product is in each package).
- What to do if an overdose occurs.

Figure J-1 is an example of the OTC "Drug Facts" section.

Drug Facts

Active ingredient (in each tablet)	**Purpose**
Chlorpheniramine maleate 2 mg	Antihistamine

Uses temporarily relieves these symptoms due to hay fever or other upper respiratory allergies: ■ sneezing ■ runny nose ■ itchy, watery eyes ■ itchy throat

Warnings

Ask a doctor before use if you have
■ glaucoma ■ a breathing problem such as emphysema or chronic bronchitis
■ trouble urinating due to an enlarged prostate gland

Ask a doctor or pharmacist before use if you are taking tranquilizers or sedatives

When using this product
■ drowsiness may occur ■ avoid alcoholic drinks
■ alcohol, sedatives, and tranquilizers may increase drowsiness
■ be careful when driving a motor vehicle or operating machinery
■ excitability may occur, especially in children

If pregnant or breast-feeding, ask a health professional before use.
Keep out of reach of children. In case of overdose, get medical help or contact a Poison Control Center right away.

Directions

adults and children 12 years and over	take 2 tablets every 4 to 6 hours; not more than 12 tablets in 24 hours
children 6 years to under 12 years	take 1 tablet every 4 to 6 hours; not more than 6 tablets in 24 hours
children under 6 years	ask a doctor

Drug Facts (continued)

Other information ■ store at 20-25° C (68-77° F) ■ protect from excessive moisture

Inactive ingredients D&C yellow no. 10, lactose, magnesium stearate, microcrystalline cellulose, pregelatinized starch

Figure J-1. Example of new Drug Facts section of nonprescription product labeling.

FDA Adverse Event Reporting System (FAERS)

The FDA Adverse Event Reporting System (FAERS) is a database that contains information on adverse event and medication error reports submitted to FDA. The database is designed to support the FDA's post-marketing safety surveillance program for drug and therapeutic biologic products.

Reporting of adverse events and medication errors by health

care professionals and consumers is voluntary in the United States. FDA receives some adverse event and medication error reports directly from health care professionals (such as physicians, pharmacists, nurses and others) and consumers (such as patients, family members, lawyers and others). Health care professionals and consumers may also report adverse events and/or medication errors to the products' manufacturers. If a manufacturer receives an adverse event report, it is required to send the report to FDA. The reports received directly and the reports from manufacturers are entered into the FAERS system.

FAERS is a useful tool for FDA for activities such as looking for new safety concerns that might be related to a marketed product, evaluating a manufacturer's compliance to reporting regulations and responding to outside requests for information. The reports in FAERS are evaluated by clinical reviewers in the Center for Drug Evaluation and Research (CDER) and the Center for Biologics Evaluation and Research (CBER) to monitor the safety of products after they are approved by FDA. If a potential safety concern is identified in FAERS, further evaluation is performed. Based on an evaluation of the potential safety concern, FDA may take regulatory action(s) to improve product safety and protect the public health, such as updating a product's labeling information, restricting the use of the drug, communicating new safety information to the public, or, in rare cases, removing a product from the market.

OTC Labeling for Pregnancy and Nursing Mothers

Federal regulations mandate labeling for nonprescription drug products intended for systemic use. The general warning states: "As with any drug, if you are pregnant or nursing a baby, seek the advice of a health professional before using this product". Exceptions to this labeling will include those drugs intended to benefit the fetus or nursing infant and those products intended exclusively for pediatric use.

Some OTC drugs, such as oral or rectal products containing aspirin, must have the warning: "It is especially important not to use this product during the last three months of pregnancy unless specifically directed to do so by a doctor".

OTC Labeling of Sodium Content

Federal regulations require that the labeling for OTC products intended for oral administration must indicate the sodium content per dosage unit (i.e., per teaspoonful, tablespoonful, etc.), if the amount present exceeds 5 mg per single dose. This total refers to all sources of sodium whether present in active or inactive ingredients.

If the amount of sodium present in the labeled maximum daily dose of the product is more than 140 milligrams, a warning on the label must state: "Ask a doctor before use if you have a sodium-restricted diet".

Acceptable terminology indicating sodium levels is specified in Figure J-2.

DESIGNATION	MEANING
Sodium Free	Contains 5 mg or less of sodium in the labeled maximum daily dose
Very Low Sodium	Contains 35 mg or less of sodium in the labeled maximum daily dose
Low Sodium	Contains 140 mg or less of sodium in the lableled maximum daily dose

Figure J-2. Meaning of OTC Sodium Level Designations

Note

All of the above quantities refer to the content of sodium, NOT sodium chloride.

The labeling of OTC drug products intended for rectal administration containing dibasic sodium phosphate and/or monobasic sodium phosphate must contain the sodium content per delivered dose if the sodium content is 5 milligrams or more.

OTC Labeling for Other Electrolytes

In 2004, the FDA issued rules for labeling other electrolytes present in OTC products. The label must indicate the presence of each of the following minerals if the level of the mineral in each dose is equal to or exceeds the threshold amount indicated:

Mineral	Threshold Amount
Calcium	20 mg
Magnesium	8 mg
Potassium	5 mg

In addition, label warnings intended for individuals on electrolyte-restricted diets are required if the maximum daily intake of a mineral will exceed the threshold amounts indicated below.

Mineral	Threshold Amount
Sodium	140 mg
Calcium	3.2 g
Magnesium	600 mg
Potassium	975 mg

Tamper-resistant Packaging Act

After several instances of deliberate addition of poisons to commercial nonprescription drug packages on store shelves, the Tamper-resistant Packaging Act was passed. The intent of this Act is to prevent the intentional contamination of over-the-counter products.

Some exemptions from the requirement include:

- aerosol products.
- nonprescription products not accessible to the general public (such as those in hospitals and other institutions).
- lozenges, and drugs in first aid kits.

In November 1998, the Act was clarified by using the term "Tamper-evident Packaging". It is intended to heighten consumer awareness of potential tampering, without implying that a particular package is difficult to open or that it is "tamper- proof".

This legislation also requires that two-piece hard gelatin capsules must be sealed using a tamper-evident technology and that the packages containing the capsules have at least one tamper-evident feature.

Medicaid Tamper-Resistant Prescription Requirement

In 2008 the Centers for Medicare & Medicaid Services (CMS) issued a requirement that specified that all written, non-electronic prescriptions for Medicaid outpatient drugs that were to be reimbursable by the federal government must contain at least three tamper-resistant features. They must be designed to

- prevent unauthorized copying of a completed or blank prescription form;
- prevent the erasure or modification of information written on the prescription by the prescriber
- prevent the use of counterfeit prescription forms.

The tamper-resistant requirement does not apply to durable medical equipment, prosthetics, orthotics, and supplies such as diabetic testing strips?

Since the individual states are responsible for implementing Medicaid regulations, each state Medicaid Agency has issued its own guidance on this requirement. In preparing for the MPJE®, candidates are advised to become aware of these state requirements.

Prescription to OTC Reclassification

Requests for the reclassification of a prescription-only drug to OTC status are accomplished by one of the following four mechanisms:

- If the drug is now a prescription drug, a full NDA (New Drug Application) requesting OTC status may be submitted to the FDA for its evaluation.
- The FDA may grant an exemption if it deems that prescription-only status is unnecessary for the protection of the public health.
- A supplement to the NDA may be filed. The FDA will then review the relative safety of the drug based upon previous marketing experience and lack of a history of adverse effects.
- The Nonprescription Drug Advisory Committee may recommend that a particular ingredient be converted to nonprescription status.

The Nonprescription Drug Advisory Committees were originally established to evaluate the numerous nonprescription products and individual ingredients currently on the market. The committees or panels, subdivided by therapeutic categories, submitted their conclusions to the FDA. As a result of their deliberations, OTC ingredients were classified into one of three categories.

- **Category I** - Generally recognized as safe and effective (GRASE) for the claimed therapeutic indication.
- **Category II** - Not generally recognized as safe and effective or having unacceptable indications.
- **Category III** - Insufficient data available to permit final classification.

Based upon data submitted or following the failure of companies to submit data, the status of specific OTC ingredients may be changed from one category to another. For example, in 2002, the FDA banned the use of aloe and cascara sagrada as laxative ingredients in over-the-counter drug products. These two groups of ingredients are deemed as not being GRASE (generally recognized as safe and effective). This effectively placed these ingredients into Category II. Laxative products containing any form of aloe or cascara sagrada are, therefore, now considered to be misbranded.

> **Note**
>
> Questions on either the NAPLEX® or the MPJE® may be designed to determine if the candidate is familiar with the status of a specific drug product. Drugs or drug products that were switched from Rx-only to nonprescription status within the past few years may be included. However, the exam will likely avoid including drug products whose status may change in the near future or those that are being presently evaluated for a change. It is unlikely that questions that ask for concentrations or strengths of prescription versus nonprescription products will be asked on the MPJE®.

Refilling Prescriptions Written for Nonprescription Drugs

The pharmacist may refill prescriptions written for nonprescription drugs without prescriber authorization unless:

1. The dose requested is greater than the recommended dose on the label of the commercial OTC product.
2. The prescriber has limited the number of refills on the original prescription.
3. The drug is a Schedule V controlled substance where the number of refills must be designated by the prescriber.
4. The individual state has set a time period limit for refills.

Sample Questions

1. A physician writes prescription for a nonprescription drug with no refill instructions. The pharmacist:

   (A) may NOT refill the prescription

   (B) may refill only once

   (C) may refill at his/her discretion

   (D) must contact the physician before refilling

   (E) should supply a one day supply of drug

2. Manufacturers would most fear the reclassification of their nonprescription product from category

   (A) I to II (B) II to I (C) I to III

   (D) III to I (E) II to III

3. The levels of all of the following electrolytes must be listed on OTC labels EXCEPT

   (A) calcium (B) chloride (C) magnesium

   (D) potassium (E) sodium

4. The preferred term for packaging that helps prevent contamination of nonprescription drug products is:

   (A) child-proof (B) occlusive (C) poison-prevention

   (D) tamper-evident (E) tamper-proof

5. All of the following are exempt from tamper-evident packaging requirements EXCEPT

   (A) aerosols

   (B) drugs in first-aid kits

   (C) 2-piece hard gelatin capsules

   (D) 1-piece hard gelatin capsules

   (E) no exceptions

Answers:

(1) C (2) A (3) B (4) D (5) C

Section K

Dietary and Nutritional Supplements

Dietary Supplement Health Education Act (DSHEA)

DSHEA places health foods, food supplements, and herbal products into a class different from prescription and nonprescription drugs. Included in the class are herbals, amino acids, vitamins, minerals, and related supplements. Among the major provisions of the original act and later additions are:

- Products may be marketed without their efficacy proven. The FDA or FTC would have to challenge products after they had been introduced onto the market if evidence surfaced that they are ineffective for the advertised or labeled use.
- Products currently on the market do not have to be proven safe. It is the responsibility of the FDA to prove that a product is unsafe. However, the manufacturer must provide "reasonable" assurances that no ingredient in the product presents a significant or unreasonable risk for illness or injury.
- The USP has published the "Manufacturing Practices for Dietary Supplements" in USP General Chapter 2750. Effective in 2007, the FDA regulations for Good Manufacturing Practices (GMP's) for dietary supplements were published. These regulations make distinctions between:

  A. Dietary Supplement (DS) - i.e. the final Product.

  B. Dietary Ingredient (DI) - i.e. a vitamin, mineral, herb or other botanical, an amino acid, or a dietary substance to supplement the diet.

  C. Non-DI - i.e. an excipient or substance used in the manufacture of a DS.

The complete definition in the Federal Food, Drug and Cosmetic Act reads: "A dietary ingredient is a vitamin, mineral, herb, or other botanical, amino acid, a dietary substance to supplement the diet by increasing the total dietary intake, or a concentrate, metabolite, constituent, extract, or combination of any of the aforementioned ingredients".

Under this Act, most of the new requirements fall upon the manufacturer of the dietary supplement with respect to testing and record-keeping. The GMP rules do not provide specific guidelines or requirements for tests that a company needs to conduct to verify identity, purity, strength, and composition of ingredients and finished products. Instead, the company may establish its own testing procedures. Also the company could either test every batch of finished products or a subset of finished batches. The company may perform tests on the non-DI or it may rely on a Certificate of Analysis (C of A) obtained from the supplier of the non-DI.

The manufacturers must establish and follow written procedures for their operations and facilities. They must keep written product records for one year past the expiration date (if such a date has been determined,) or two years beyond the date of distribution of the last batch of supplements.

Suppliers of dietary ingredients are not required to conform to the new GMP rules since the responsibility of determining DI quality belongs with the manufacturer of the finished DS product. The exception occurs when a company manufactures a DI that is then simply repackaged as a final product. In these cases, the company is subjected to the GMP rules.

Violations of the GMP rules will result in the product being considered "adulterated".

Official Status of Herbals

The *USP/NF* has developed monographs for some botanicals that appear to have therapeutic efficiency. To be admitted into the official compendium, the herb must have an FDA approved use or a *USP DI* Panel recognized use. The monographs describe the portion of plant used, its botanical characteristics, and appropriate assay procedure for ingredients. The monographs do not describe the therapeutic use of the herbs. Among the herbs with monographs are chamomile, cranberry liquid preparations, feverfew, garlic, ginger, ginkgo, milk thistle, St John's wort, saw palmetto, and valerian.

Labeling for Herbals and Dietary Supplements

Labels for herbal products must contain the standard common names as listed in the reference source, *Herbs of Commerce*, published by the AHPA (American Herbal Products Association). This reference source contains standardized common herbal names as well as corresponding Latin binomial designations for thousands of herbal species. In 2006 this publication was incorporated officially into federal regulations for the labeling of botanical ingredients in dietary supplements. The standardized common herbal names must be used, but inclusion of the Latin names is optional. For example, the name of Eleuthero for the herb *Eleutherococcus senticosus* must be used rather than "Siberian ginseng". If an herb is not listed in the *Herbs of Commerce*, the manufacturer must include the herb's Latin name on the label.

Manufacturers are permitted to make structure or function claims on labels if the statements do not indicate that the product will diagnose, cure, treat, or prevent a disease. Some claims related to the product's ability to affect body structure or function are permitted if they are truthful and not misleading. For example, a claim that saw palmetto will "improve urinary flow" or that it is "for the prostate" is acceptable. However, a statement that it "will cure or reduce the size of an enlarged prostate" is not acceptable. While the manufacturer must substantiate the product claims, they do NOT have to be reviewed or approved by the FDA. This fact must be stated on the product label. Often the warning will read, "These claims have not been evaluated by the Food and Drug Administration. This product is not intended to diagnose, treat, cure, or prevent any disease."

An additional term that may lead to confusion is **nutraceuticals**, which may be defined as food products including dietary supplements, herbals, and processed foods that provide health or medical benefits, including prevention or treatment of diseases.

> ***Note***
>
> Since there is an ongoing dialogue between the FDA and manufacturers of the above products as to the interpretation of allowable claims, it is unlikely that any specific questions about these products will appear on the MPJE®.

Ban on Sales of Ephedra and Ephedrine Alkaloids

For centuries ephedra has been used for several indications including asthma. However, in 2004 the FDA banned the sales of all dietary supplements containing this drug, citing that its use posed an unreasonable risk of illness or injury to consumers. Based upon the DSHEA (Dietary Supplement Health and Education Act), the FDA claimed that dietary supplements containing ephedra or its alkaloids are adulterated since they present an unreasonable risk of illness or injury based upon their recommended use. The ban does not apply to prescription or nonprescription drug products or to conventional foods such as herbal teas. It also does not apply to products that are prepared or used for "Traditional Chinese Medicine" since this practice uses ephedra for temporary respiratory conditions, not for chronic, long-term use for weight loss. In addition, the product labels must not have any indication that the product is a dietary supplement.

Sample Questions

Answer the first four questions using the key of:

(A) I only (B) III only (C) I & II only
(D) II & III only (E) I, II, & III

1. Which of the following statements is (are) true?
   I. Commercial herbals are categorized as dietary supplements.
   II. Commercial herbals may be categorized as nonprescription drugs.
   III. None of the herbals used in the US are recognized in the *USP/NF.*

2. A pharmacist may sell herbals provided that:
   I. the patient is properly counseled with respect to their use.
   II. the consumer is cautioned to use the product for not more than two weeks.
   III. there are adequate directions on the package for patient use.

3. Upon formal request, to whom must the manufacturer of an herbal product submit data supporting the claims for the product?
   I. FDA or FTC
   II. pharmacists
   III. consumers

4. Ephedra may still be found in which of the following products?
   I. prescription drug products
   II. non-prescription drug products
   III. dietary supplements

5. Nomenclature for herbals is primarily based upon which one of the following reference sources?
   (A) Herbs of Commerce
   (B) Homeopathic Pharmacopoeia
   (C) German Commission on Herbs of Choice
   (D) USP
   (E) USP/NF
6. A practitioner of "Traditional Chinese Medicine" may sell ephedra-containing products if:
   (A) a prescription is presented.
   (B) there is no label claim that the product is a dietary supplement.
   (C) the customer is examined by the seller.
   (D) less than a 10 day supply is sold.
   (E) the product is marked for long-term use for weight loss

Answers:

(1) A (2) B (3) A (4) C (5) A (6) B

Homeopathic Drug Products

The Federal Food, Drug and Cosmetic Act of 1938 recognized the *Homeopathic Pharmacopoeia of the United States (HPUS)* as an official compendium. Drug products that use an official name designation found in the *HPUS* must meet all of its compendial standards. Otherwise the drug product is misbranded or adulterated.

The basic elements of homeopathic medicine include individualized dosing of patients by homeopathic physicians, based upon a patient's symptoms. The dose of drug administered is usually extremely low; often dilutions of 1:1,000 or 1:1,000,000 are used with frequent drug administration. These drug products must meet the usual drug labeling requirements including ingredient names, amounts, and directions for use. While many of the drugs were originally labeled by their Latin name, it is now required that their English name be provided. Some of the drugs found in homeopathic formulas are also official in the *USP/NF*. In these situations, the drug must meet the stricter standards found in the *USP/NF*. If the drug product is intended for nonprescription use, its label must include appropriate warning statements, if needed.

While homeopathic drugs must be manufactured under GMP standards, they do not have to have an expiration date on their package.

Section L

Cosmetics

The legal distinction between cosmetics and drugs is somewhat muddled. For example, some cosmetics, such as fluoridated toothpaste, medicated mouthwash, or anti-dandruff shampoos are on the borderline between being classified as cosmetics or as non-prescription products. The overriding factor in determining a product's status may not be its ingredients, but what claims are made for the product, especially on the label. Unlike drugs, cosmetics do not require premarketing approval from the FDA.

While cosmetic manufacturers do not have to meet the rigorous requirements of the FDA's Good Manufacturing Practice (GMP) program, they are still obligated to manufacture these products under sanitary conditions. Otherwise, the products could be considered to be adulterated. While the Federal Food, Drug, and Cosmetic Act of 1938 does not specifically state that cosmetics have to be tested for safety, any cosmetic that poses a safety problem to the general public will be considered as being misbranded. If an unapproved color additive is used in the formulation, the product will be classified as being adulterated.

Regulation of advertising and labeling of cosmetics basically falls under the jurisdiction of the Federal Trade Commission (FTC). The labels of cosmetic products must contain the names of ingredients listed in descending order of predominance (that is why water may be listed as the first ingredient, while the "active ingredient" is listed further down in the ingredient list). Ingredients present in quantities of one percent or less may be listed at the bottom, in random order. Perfumes and flavoring oils may simply be listed by name. Coloring agents must be those accepted for cosmetic use. A minor exception to the above ingredient-listing requirement is cosmetics used in professional settings such as by professional hairdressers (i.e. cosmetics not intended for retail sales).

The ingredient names listed on labels must be the generic names listed in the *USP/NF*. If an ingredient is not of *USP/NF* quality or is not listed in these two official books, other relevant sources such as the *CTFA Cosmetic Ingredient Dictionary* may be used. This book has been compiled by the Cosmetic, Toiletry, and Fragrance Association (CTFA) and contains many ingredients commonly used in cosmetics (e.g. surfactants).

Many cosmetic products, especially those intended for use in body cavities (e.g. mouthwashes and vaginal products), must be packaged in tamper-resistant packaging.

Sunscreen Innovation Act (2014)

The approval of new ingredients for sunscreen products has been very slow in the past. This act requires the FDA to respond quickly to requests for approval of pending ingredients for OTC sunscreen products.

Sample Questions

1. Which one of the following organizations is responsible for establishing names for ingredients used in cosmetic formulations?

   (A) ASHP (B) AHPA (C) CTFA
   (D) HCFA (E) RDA

2. A client in a pharmacy complains about her hypersensitivity to many ingredients found in cosmetic lotions. When reading the label of a sunscreen lotion, which one of the following ingredients is not required to be listed by the manufacturer?

   (A) antimicrobial preservative (B) coloring agent
   (C) sunscreen agent (D) perfuming oil
   (E) water

3. The general guideline for listing ingredients on a cosmetic product label consists of listing the additives

(A) and active ingredients intermixed but in the alphabetical sequence.

(B) and active ingredients intermixed but ranked by decreasing concentrations.

(C) and active ingredients intermixed but ranked by increasing concentrations.

(D) separately from the active ingredients by increasing concentration.

(E) separately from the active ingredients by decreasing concentrations.

4. A cosmetic hand lotion consists of an oil-in-water emulsion. The first ingredient listed on its label is most likely to be the:

(A) oil that is present
(B) water
(C) coloring agent
(D) surfactant
(E) perfume

5. Which one of the following is the basic goal for the 2014 Sunscreen Innovation Act?

(A) speed the marketing of new sunscreen products
(B) speed the approval of new sunscreen ingredients
(C) establish a newcode for screen efficacy
(D) provide funds for developing new sunscreen ingredients
(E) reduce the cost of sunscreen products

Answers:

(1) C (2) D (3) B (4) B (5) B

Section M

Miscellaneous Laws and Regulations

Alcohol Regulations

The Bureau of Alcohol, Tobacco and Firearms controls the sale of alcohol. Pharmacies may purchase 95% ethanol (190 proof grain alcohol) for routine compounding by using Form ATF-11. If a pharmacy is selling alcohol in the form of a beverage, it must obtain a retail liquor dealer's stamp. Institutions that have a need for greater volumes of alcohol may choose to purchase tax-free alcohol, since it is much lower in cost (tax on regular alcohol purchases is very high). Such pharmacies must purchase alcohol by using Form ATF-1447.

The following are federal statutes that relate to the use of tax-free alcohol:

- Its use is limited to medicinal or scientific use, or in patient treatment.
- The alcohol may not be sold or loaned to other pharmacies or physician's offices.
- The alcohol, either by itself or as a component of other products, may not be sold to outpatients. An exception to this requirement permits nonprofit clinics to dispense medicines made with tax-free alcohol provided the client is not charged for the medication.
- A running, accurate inventory must be kept for all alcohol in stock.
- Containers of alcohol, usually supplied in 10 or 55-gallon drums, must be stored in a securely locked, fire-resistant storeroom.

How may a prescriber's order for an alcohol-containing beverage (e.g. brandy at bedtime) for an institutionalized client be handled? Either the

- institution may buy the alcohol-containing beverage, furnish it to the client, and then bill the patient, or
- the hospital pharmacy may give the patient's relatives permission to bring in alcohol for the patient.

Another available form of tax-exempt alcohol is Specially Denatured Alcohol (SDA). SDAs refer to specific formulas of grain (ethyl) alcohol that have been rendered unsuitable for use as a beverage by the addition of denaturants such as sucrose octaacetate, brucine, or butyl alcohol. There are a large number of formulas for SDAs, usually designated as SDA 40A, SDA 23H, etc. SDAs are often used for pharmaceutical processing and in commercial products such as mouthwashes.

Americans with Disabilities Act (ADA)

The Federal Rehabilitation Act of 1973 prevents an employer from discriminating against a person who is physically or mentally handicapped, but who is otherwise qualified to perform the functions of a job. The Act applies only to those companies receiving federal assistance.

The Americans with Disabilities Act (ADA) became effective in 1992. This Act expands the original Rehabilitation Act by greatly increasing the number of individuals covered and by covering companies even if they are not receiving federal financial assistance. Any company employing 15 or more people is covered. In both acts, the term "disabled" is used since it has less of a negative connotation than the term "handicapped".

These acts provide civil rights protection to individuals with disabilities similar to those provided to individuals on the basis of race, color, sex, national origin, age, and religion. Among those covered under the ADA are individuals with epilepsy, paralysis, HIV infections, AIDS, mental retardation, and alcoholics. Those NOT protected are individuals who illegally use drugs. A key concept of both acts is that employers must make a "reasonable effort" to accommodate a disabled employee.

The following are additional elements of these laws:

- The employer must make reasonable accommodations for disabled individuals whether those individuals are employees or members of the general public. For the general public, "reasonable accommodations" include providing ramps leading into a building, providing elevator service to all floors of a building, and constructing restroom facilities that are accessible to disabled individuals.
- For an employee, "reasonable accommodations" might include a reduced-height workbench.
- An employer may not ask about disabilities during an employment interview, but may ask if the prospective employee has the ability to perform the work.

> **Note**
>
> A court has ruled that pharmacists who are HIV positive may not be discriminated against by either refusing them employment or by refusing to assign them to the usual daily functions of a pharmacist. This concept could be extended to pregnant female pharmacists who may wish to prepare chemotherapy drug admixtures. Obviously if they prefer NOT to work with potentially mutagenic agents, their wishes should be honored.

- An employer may not require a prospective employee to undergo a medical examination before offering a position. However, the employer may require a medical examination as a condition of employment if this is a requirement for all new employees.

> **Note**
>
> Tests for illegal use of drugs are not considered to be medical examinations and may be required by an employer.

Sample Questions

1. The requirements of the ADA must be followed if what minimum number of employees is employed in a pharmacy?

   (A) 2 (B) 10 (C) 15 (D) 50 (E) 100

2. Which of the following conditions may preclude a pharmacist from working in a hospital pharmacy?

   I. alcoholism
   II. HIV infection
   III. cocaine addiction

   (A) I only (B) III only (C) I & II only
   (D) II & III only (E) I, II, & III

3. An institutional pharmacy employer may NOT prevent pharmacists with which of the following conditions from working in a parenteral admixture room?

   I. chronic alcoholism
   II. HIV infection
   III. epilepsy

   (A) I only (B) III only (C) I & II only
   (D) II & III only (E) I, II, & III

4. The ADA protects an employee if an employer attempts to enforce:

I. random locker room searches for illegal drugs

II. IQ tests

III. weight reduction programs

(A) I only (B) III only (C) I & II only

(D) II & III only (E) I, II, & III

Answers: (1) C (2) B (3) E (4) D

E-mail use in Pharmacy Practice

A federal law passed in December 2003, sometimes called the CAN-SPAM act, affects all unsolicited commercial e-mailing. The law's intent is to reduce unsolicited e-mailing (i.e. spam) from all sources. All companies that issue e-mail messages must identify themselves within the message and provide physical address contact information. In addition, the subject line of the e-mail must be truthful and not deceptive.

Other requirements of this law specify that each commercial e-mail message must:

- identify itself as an advertisement or solicitation.
- originate from a legitimate e-mail address to which a recipient may reply.
- be sent from a legitimate domain name and have correct header information that allows tracing to its origin.
- have a mechanism by which a recipient may choose not to receive future messages.

An added incentive for complying with the CAN-SPAM act is that the federal government is empowered to levy a fine of up to $16,000 for each separate e-mail violation of this law.

Drug-free Workplace

According to the Federal Anti-Drug Abuse Act of 1988

- The unlawful possession of controlled substances by employees is prohibited in the workplace.
- If an employee is convicted of criminal possession of drugs, he/she must inform the employer of the conviction within five days.
- Employers may take appropriate action.

Unfair Competition

It is unlikely that questions concerning the economic aspects of pharmacy will be asked on the MPJE®. However, one should be aware of two major laws in this area.

Sherman Antitrust Act

The Sherman Antitrust Act prevents restraint of trade or the establishment of monopolies. Originally, the Sherman Antitrust Act was intended to curtail the large monopolies that operated in the early 1900's. The concept of the Act is to prevent restraint of trade and/or the establishment of monopolies.

Companies or groups may not have agreements, either formal or informal, among themselves, which would unreasonably restrain trade. For example, three independent pharmacies in a given area may not agree to a common drug mark-up of 40% or a professional fee of $15.00. These actions would probably be classified as price fixing. Other examples could be the distribution of suggested retail prices for certain prescription drugs by a pharmaceutical organization or the boycott by a group of pharmacies of a third party payer because of its low reimbursement rate. In addition, a group of pharmacies may not agree as a group to reject a third-party prescription plan, nor can they collectively bargain for better reimbursement rates. However, a chain consisting of several pharmacies may do so.

Robinson-Patman Act

The intent of the Robinson-Patman Act is to prevent the hindering of competition. A seller is not allowed to practice price discrimination when dealing with similar purchasers. For example, the wholesale price for 100 x 1,000 tablet bottles may not favor one pharmacy over another. Likewise, this issue arises when individual states allow hospitals to dispense prescriptions for walk-in clients if the hospital has a community pharmacy permit. In this case, however, the price of the prescription may not be based upon the special, reduced price that the hospital receives from the pharmaceutical manufacturer. Nor can the hospital sell drugs or medical devices to affiliated groups such as a home health care business at the special, reduced price.

Hospitals and similar institutions do have the right to extend their special prices to employees, inpatients, emergency room patients, etc. This is known as "own use". Institutions are not permitted to provide prescription refills for former patients unless the take-home drugs are intended as continued care or are supplementing treatment administered in the hospital (e.g. continuing a treatment with parenteral antibiotics).

While physicians on the hospital staff may be supplied with drugs for personal use, drugs may not be sold to physicians for use in their private practice, especially if the drugs are being sold to patients.

Section N

Sample Questions

1. In which of the following situations are child-resistant closures required?
   - I. When a community pharmacist dispenses fewer than 10 tablets of a drug product
   - II. When a hospital pharmacy fills a prescription for an outpatient
   - III. When a hospital pharmacy fills a prescription for an inpatient

   (A) I only (B) III only (C) I & II only
   (D) II & III only (E) I, II, & III

2. Permission to omit the use a child-resistant closure when filling a prescription may be granted by the
   - I. patient
   - II. prescriber
   - III. pharmacist

   (A) I only (B) III only (C) I & II only
   (D) II & III only (E) I, II, & III

3. The Marketing Act of 1987 guarantees a company that discovers, patents, and develops a new drug exclusive marketing rights for up to:

   (A) 50 years (B) 20 years (C) 17 years
   (D) 10 years (E) 100 years

4. Auto injectors are commercially available for the administration of
   (A) naloxone
   (B) hydrochlorthiazide
   (C) amlodipine
   (D) certraline
   (E) gabapentin
5. Which of the following reference sources include selected laws and regulations for controlled substances?
   (A) Facts and Comparisons
   (B) Physician's Desk Reference
   (C) USP DI Volume I
   (D) USP DI Volume II
   (E) USP DI Volume III
6. When listing an ingredient on a product label, all of the following references may be used by manufacturers as primary sources for names EXCEPT.
   (A) CTFA Cosmetic Ingredient Dictionary
   (B) USAN
   (C) Food Chemicals Codex
   (D) Facts and Comparisons
   (E) USP Dictionary of Drug Names
7. Which one of the following incentives is used to encourage pharmaceutical companies to conduct studies of their drugs in the pediatric population?
   (A) extension of patent protection
   (B) tax credits for subsequent years
   (C) refunds of income tax
   (D) grants of money from the FDA
   (E) fewer visits from the FDA

8. Under which one of the following circumstances may a pharmacist refuse to fill a prescription?
   (A) The prescriber is from another city.
   (B) The pharmacist does not know the patient.
   (C) The patient is an alcoholic.
   (D) The prescription was written a week ago.
   (E) The quantity of the controlled drug has been changed.

9. The drug patent of an innovator company has expired. Which one of the following must a second drug company submit to place a generic form of the drug product onto the market?
   (A) Abbreviated new drug application
   (B) Investigational new drug application
   (C) New drug application
   (D) Generic drug application
   (E) Supplemental new drug application

10. The term "donut hole" refers to a component of which one of the following?
   (A) Medicare Part B
   (B) National Drug Code
   (C) Medicare Part D
   (D) Poison Prevention Act
   (E) Prescription Drug Marketing Act of 1987

11. Into how many segments is the NDC number on a pharmaceutical package divided?
   (A) 5 (B) 2 (C) 4
   (D) 3 (E) 7

12. Which of the following barbiturates are classified as Schedule II controlled substances?

    I. butabarbital

    II. pentobarbital

    III. amobarbital

    (A) I only (B) III only (C) I & II only
    (D) II & III only (E) I, II, & III

13. Which one of the following reference sources is the most appropriate choice when a manufacturer is determining the preferred name of an additive for a product label?

    (A) CTFA *Cosmetic Ingredient Dictionary*
    (B) *Food Chemicals Codex*
    (C) USAN
    (D) *USP Dictionary of Drug Names*
    (E) USP/NF

14. Which of the following drug products must be ordered using DEA Form 222?

    I. Fentanyl

    II. Vicodin

    III. Pentobarbital

    (A) I only (B) III only (C) I & II only
    (D) II & III only (E) I, II, & III

15. Which government body is responsible for funding and overseeing state Medicaid programs?

    (A) DHHS (B) CMS (C) FDA
    (D) NABP (E) USP/NF

16. Which of the following clinical trial stages is conducted exclusively in healthy humans?

    (A) phase I (B) phase II (C) phase III
    (D) phase IV (E) phase I and II

17. The first phase of a clinical trial, which evaluates the efficacy of the drug in treating a specific disease, is:

(A) phase I (B) phase II (C) phase III
(D) phase IV (E) phase V

18. Under which of the following conditions may a pharmaceutical sales representative distribute samples of a prescription drug product?

I. Upon written request from a physician
II. Upon written request from a hospital pharmacy
III. Upon written request from a community pharmacy

(A) I only (B) III only (C) I & II only
(D) II & III only (E) I, II, & III

19. Which of the following may a nurse in a doctor's office perform, with the prescriber's permission, with regard to a Schedule III prescription?

I. write the prescription and sign prescriber's name
II. write the prescription except for the drug name, strength, quantity and prescriber's name
III. write the entire prescription except for signing the prescriber's name

(A) I only (B) III only (C) I & II only
(D) II & III only (E) I, II, & III

20. After dispensing prescriptions for several months for a Schedule II analgesic, the pharmacist realizes that the patient with severe pain from malignant bone cancer is addicted to the drug. Which one of the following actions is the most appropriate for the pharmacist?

(A) Report the situation to the state board of pharmacy.
(B) Report the situation to the state medical board.
(C) Report the situation to the DEA.
(D) Refuse to fill any further prescriptions.
(E) Continue to fill the prescriptions.

21. How frequently may a patient with a Medicare-endorsed discount card change his/her provider?
    (A) every month
    (B) every 6 months
    (C) whenever he/she desires
    (D) once a year
    (E) never

22. A pharmacist may fill prescriptions for and mail which of the following drugs through the US Postal Service?
    I. Schedule II non-narcotics
    II. Benzodiazepines
    III. Schedule II narcotics
    (A) I only (B) III only (C) I & II only
    (D) II & III only (E) I, II, & III

23. The selling of drug samples in pharmacies is prohibited by which one of the following Federal acts?
    (A) DSHEA
    (B) Durham Humphrey Amendment
    (C) Prescription Drug Marketing Act
    (D) Sherman Act
    (E) Drug Price Competition Act

24. In 2002, the FDA ruled that the nonprescription drug ingredient, cascara sagrada, belongs in the OTC Category II. Products containing this ingredient will be considered by the FDA to be
    (A) adulterated
    (B) misbranded
    (C) safe and effective
    (D) potentially toxic
    (E) expired

25. Who is responsible for the retrospective drug utilization reviews established by OBRA 90?
    (A) each state
    (B) consultant pharmacists
    (C) individual community pharmacies
    (D) hospital pharmacies
    (E) all dispensing pharmacists

26. HCFA is under the jurisdiction of the
    (A) Attorney General (B) HHS
    (C) JCAHO (D) FDA
    (E) Dept. of Justice

27. A pharmacist who fills an oral morphine sulfate prescription in an emergency does not receive a "cover" prescription from the prescriber. The pharmacist must
    I. notify the regional DEA office.
    II. notify the state board of medicine.
    III. call the patient and request that he/she obtain a written prescription to cover the oral order.
    (A) I only (B) III only (C) I & II only
    (D) II & III only (E) I, II, & III

28. A patient presents a prescription for 60 Tylenol w/codeine tablets No.4 to his local pharmacy and indicates that he would only like to get 30 of the tablets now and will return for the other 30 in a week. The pharmacist should
    (A) call the prescriber to get permission to dispense 30
    (B) dispense 30 tablets as requested by the patient.
    (C) advise the patient that the full 60 tablets must be supplied at one time.
    (D) fill the prescription as requested by the patient but advise the patient that the balance must be picked up within 72 hours.
    (E) dispense 30 tabs of Tylenol w/codeine No. 2

29. Which of the following reference book(s) are legal documents recognized by the federal government?

    I. USP/NF

    II. Homeopathic Pharmacopeia of the U.S.

    III. Remington's Pharmaceutical Sciences

    (A) I only (B) III only (C) I & II only

    (D) II & III only (E) I, II, & III

30. Which of the following conditions must exist for the inspection of a pharmacy by an authorized inspector?

    I. The inspector must have a search warrant.

    II. The owner of the pharmacy or the designated supervising pharmacist must be present.

    III. Inspection must be conducted during the regular business hours of the pharmacy.

    (A) I only (B) III only (C) I & II only

    (D) II & III only (E) I, II, & III

31. Schedule III, IV, or V controlled substances may be refilled

    I. not more than 6 times

    II. not more than for a 6 month period

    III. only if authorized by the prescriber

    (A) I only (B) III only (C) I & II only

    (D) II & III only (E) I, II, & III

32. Which of the following are mid-level practitioners?

    I. Dermatologist

    II. Nurse Midwives

    III. Nurse Practitioners

    (A) I only (B) III only (C) I & II only

    (D) II & III only (E) I, II, & III

33. A pharmacist who does not receive a registration renewal form from DEA within 45 days before the expiration of his/her registration must notify

I. the DEA in writing and request renewal forms

II. the regional FDA office

III. his/her state's board of pharmacy

(A) I only (B) III only (C) I & II only

(D) II & III only (E) I, II, & III

34. A pharmacist telephones a patient's home to remind her of an upcoming refill. With which of the following parties may the message be left?

I. patient's husband

II. patient's mother

III. patient's brother-in-law

(A) I only (B) III only (C) I & II only

(D) II & III only (E) I, II, & III

35. A pharmacist dispenses a refill for a prescription that originally was written for Adalat but labels the refill as Procardia. This action may be considered:

(A) adulteration

(B) misbranding

(C) misbranding since the generic name was not included

(D) proper since the correct drug was dispensed

(E) negligent only if the prescriber is not informed

36. When a Schedule II prescription is partially filled for a LTCF patient

    I. the total quantity dispensed cannot exceed 100 dosage units.

    II. the pharmacist must write "LTCF patient" on the prescription.

    III. the prescription is valid not more than 60 days from the issue date.

    (A) I only (B) III only (C) I & II only
    (D) II & III only (E) I, II, & III

37. When inspecting a chain pharmacy, a DEA inspector may audit which of the following records?

    I. financial records of prescription sales and profits

    II. invoices for controlled substances

    III. prescription files

    (A) I only (B) III only (C) I & II only
    (D) II & III only (E) I, II, & III

38. Certain drug products are exempt from the requirements of therapeutic equivalence because of:

    I. their high therapeutic index

    II. their use in chemotherapy

    III. the grandfather clause

    (A) I only (B) III only (C) I & II only
    (D) II & III only (E) I, II, & III

39. The National Drug Code (NDC) consists of a series of

    (A) letters only

    (B) letters and numbers

    (C) numbers only

    (D) numbers and symbols

    (E) symbols only

40. A pharmacist confides in his hospital's chief pharmacist that he has tested positive for HIV. Which of the following statements is(are) true?

I. The pharmacist may be considered disabled under the Americans with Disabilities Act.

II. The pharmacist's access to the preparation of parenteral admixtures may be limited.

III. The pharmacist may be terminated due to a potentially contagious condition.

(A) I only (B) III only (C) I & II only
(D) II & III only (E) I, II & III

41. Under which of the following circumstances may Ipecac Syrup be sold without a prescription?

I. if the purchaser signs a pharmacy log book for the sale

II. only if the household does not have small children

III. for future potential use during accidental poisoning

(A) I only (B) III only (C) I & II only
(D) II & III only (E) I, II, & III

42. Which of the following reference sources contain significant information concerning the bioequivalence of drug products?

I. *USP/NF*

II. *USP/DI*

III. Electronic Orange Book

(A) I only (B) III only (C) I & II only
(D) II & III only (E) I, II, & III

43. A neighboring community pharmacy requests Alcohol USP/NF from your hospital pharmacy, which has tax-free alcohol. Under what circumstances may you supply the alcohol?

(A) Any circumstances are permissible

(B) Limiting your sale to not more than one pint

(C) By making a simple loan of the alcohol

(D) By charging the pharmacy the purchase price plus the alcohol tax

(E) It is never permissible

44. Which of the following items provided by pharmaceutical companies are legal for community pharmacies to possess for the dispensing of prescription drugs?

I. Drug samples that are properly labeled

II. Vouchers intended for filling from the pharmacy's stock

III. Starter packs

(A) I only (B) III only (C) I & II only

(D) II & III only (E) I, II, & III

45. The presence of which of the following drugs or adjuvants in a commercial drug product requires a special label warning?

I. aspartame

II. sulfites

III. methylparaben

(A) I only (B) III only (C) I & II only

(D) II & III only (E) I, II, & III

46. A physician telephones a pharmacy and prescribes 40 Percodan tablets, 1 TID. Which of the following is/are true?

    I. It may only be dispensed in an emergency.

    II. A written "cover" prescription must be received before the pharmacist may dispense the medication.

    III. Not more than a 7-day supply may be prescribed orally.

    (A) I only (B) III only (C) I & II only
    (D) II & III only (E) I, II, & III

47. Which of the following drug products must be purchased by a pharmacy with the use of a DEA Form 222?

    I. OxyContin

    II. Dilaudid

    III. Marinol Capsules

    (A) I only (B) III only (C) I & II only
    (D) II & III only (E) I, II, & III

48. A pharmacy providing services under the Medicare Modernization Act of 2003, which uses the program's discount cards, may establish a formulary limiting the drugs to which of the following?

    (A) the top 200 frequently dispensed drugs
    (B) at least one drug from each of 208 therapeutic categories
    (C) only brand-name drugs
    (D) 100 brand-name drugs plus their equivalent generic products
    (E) only drugs available generically

49. Proposed regulations from the FDA are first published in the:
    (A) Federal Register
    (B) Congressional Record
    (C) The Drug Times
    (D) *USP/NF*
    (E) Supplements of the *USP/NF*

50. Based upon the Federal Anti-drug Abuse Act of 1988, a pharmacy employee who is convicted of criminal possession of illegal drugs must:
    (A) resign his/her position from a pharmacy.
    (B) begin monthly urine analysis.
    (C) volunteer to enter a drug rehabilitation program.
    (D) volunteer to perform at least 1000 hours of community service.
    (E) inform his/her employer within five days of the conviction

51. Prescription drug package inserts include all of the following types of information EXCEPT:
    (A) adverse reactions
    (B) contraindications
    (C) symptoms and treatment of overdosing
    (D) AWPs
    (E) date of most recent revision of the labeling

52. When filling a controlled substance prescription written for an outpatient by a hospital resident, it is essential that the
    I. prescribed drug is in either Schedule III or IV
    II. resident must have a DEA number
    III. hospital must have a DEA number
    (A) I only (B) III only (C) I & II only
    (D) II & III only (E) I, II, & III

53. Which of the following is true of controlled substance inventories?

   I. The registrant must keep inventory records for at least 5 years from the date performed.

   II. Controlled substance inventories must be performed annually.

   III. Inventories for schedule II controlled substances must be kept separately from all other records of the pharmacy.

   (A) I only (B) III only (C) I & II only

   (D) II & III only (E) I, II, & III

54. A "Listed Chemical" is defined by the Controlled Substances Act as any chemical that is

   (A) a controlled substance

   (B) listed in the USP/NF

   (C) used in manufacturing a controlled substance

   (D) listed in the USP DI

   (E) listed in the Electronic Orange Book

55. Which one of the following is the correct format for the listing of ingredients on a product label?

   (A) The additives and active ingredients intermixed but in alphabetical sequence.

   (B) Additives and active ingredients intermixed but ranked by decreasing concentrations.

   (C) Additives and active ingredients intermixed but ranked by increasing concentrations.

   (D) Additives listed separately from the active ingredients.

   (E) Additives listed separately by decreasing concentrations.

56. Which of the following is/are NOT required to be on a prescription for a controlled substance?

I. The date of birth of the patient

II. The date on which the prescription was signed

III. DEA number of the practitioner

(A) I only (B) III only (C) I & II only
(D) II & III only (E) I, II, & III

57. Which of the following practice settings must include bar coding on pharmaceutical products?

I. Physician offices

II. Pharmacies

III. Hospitals

(A) I only (B) III only (C) I & II only
(D) II & III only (E) I, II, & III

58. The authority for determining in which controlled substance schedule a new drug will be assigned is the

(A) Director of the FDA

(B) President of the US

(C) Director of the DEA

(D) Attorney General of the United States

(E) Director of HHS

59. Which of the following agents is an anabolic steroid?

I. nandrolone

II. betamethasone

III. mometasone

(A) I only (B) III only (C) I & II only
(D) II & III only (E) I, II, & III

60. Which of the following effervescent products are exempted from the Poison Prevention Packaging Act?

I. aspirin

II. acetaminophen

III. potassium chloride

(A) I only (B) III only (C) I & II only

(D) II & III only (E) I, II, & III

61. Which of the following is TRUE of Schedule II controlled substances?

I. They may only be dispensed by a community pharmacist pursuant to a written prescription signed by the practitioner.

II. They may be administered or dispensed by a physician without a prescription to a patient with chronic pain.

III. They may be administered by an institutional pharmacist pursuant to an order for immediate administration to the ultimate user.

(A) I only (B) III only (C) I & II only

(D) II & III only (E) I, II, & III

62. The main responsibility for oversight of OTC drug advertising rests with the

(A) *USP/NF* (B) FTC (C) HCFA

(D) CMS (E) FDA

63. Which of the following actions are appropriate when mailing a narcotic drug filled pursuant to a valid prescription?

I. Package the drug container in a plain paper outer wrapping

II. Place the warning: "Narcotic, do not open while in transit" on the outer wrapping

III. Place a fictitious return address on the outer wrapping.

(A) I only (B) III only (C) I & II only

(D) II & III only (E) I, II, & III

64. Which of the following is (are) a guideline for determining the expiration date for repackaging of a drug product by a pharmacy?

   I. Use one-half of the time remaining on the original package.

   II. Do not exceed one year from the date of packaging

   III. Do not exceed the expiration date on the original package.

   (A) I only (B) III only (C) I & II only
   (D) II & III only (E) I, II, & III

65. Controlled substances prescriptions may be issued by prescribers

   I. to prescribe controlled substances for a patient with chronic pain.

   II. to prescribe drugs to be used by a patient for narcotic detoxification

   III. to obtain controlled substances for dispensing in their office

   (A) I only (B) III only (C) I & II only
   (D) II & III only (E) I, II, & III

66. The CAN-SPAM Act deals with which of the following issues?

   (A) Receipt of excessive advertising through the US mail.

   (B) Patients who cross the border to purchase Canadian drug products.

   (C) Receiving unsolicited phone calls from Canadian pharmacies.

   (D) Improper e-mail use.

   (E) Pharmacists who provide excessive counseling to patients.

67. According to federal law, a pharmacist must include which of the following on a prescription label?

I. name of the dispensing pharmacy

II. address of the dispensing pharmacy

III. name of the dispensing pharmacist

(A) I only (B) III only (C) I & II only

(D) II & III only (E) I, II, & III

68. Mr. Hess has not picked up a prescription that was filled last week. Which of the following actions is (are) legal for the pharmacist to take?

I. call the patient at home and leave a message with his son

II. call the patient and leave a message on his home answering machine.

III. send an e-mail to the patient

(A) I only (B) III only (C) I & II only

(D) II & III only (E) I, II, & III

69. Labels of OTC products that are for systemic use must include a warning specifically intended to protect:

I. geriatric women

II. nursing women

III. pregnant women

(A) I only (B) III only (C) I & II only

(D) II & III only (E) I, II, & III

70. A drug product consisting of tablets may be declared adulterated for all of the following reasons EXCEPT:
    (A) active drug has undergone partial decomposition
    (B) does not indicate number of tablets present
    (C) contains an unapproved color additive
    (D) inactive ingredient has undergone partial decomposition
    (E) manufactured in a plant that fails to meet GMP's

71. The organization responsible for the accreditation of many health institutions such as hospitals is the:
    (A) APhA (B) ASHP (C) HHS
    (D) FTC (E) JCAHO

72. The presence of which of the following adjuvants in a commercial drug product requires a special label warning?
    (A) antioxidants
    (B) tartrazine
    (C) sodium benzoate
    (D) surfactants
    (E) artificial flavors

73. Which of the following OTC products must be in a tamper-resistant package?
    I. contact lens solution
    II. hair shampoo
    III. topical lotion
    (A) I only (B) III only (C) I & II only
    (D) II & III only (E) I, II, & III

74. A physician wishes to prescribe a schedule II controlled substance for a patient residing in a hospice. How may the prescription be conveyed to a pharmacy?

    I. By e-mail

    II. By fax

    III. As a written prescription

    (A) I only (B) III only (C) I & II only

    (D) II & III only (E) I, II, & III

75. Under which of the following circumstances may Ipecac Syrup be sold without a prescription?

    I. For future possible use during accidental poisoning.

    II. Only if the household does not have small children.

    III. For limited use in a weight-loss program.

    (A) I only (B) III only (C) I & II only

    (D) II & III only (E) I, II, & III

76. All of the following drugs fall into the category of "Grandfathered Drugs" EXCEPT:

    (A) thyroid (B) ephedrine

    (C) ampicillin (D) phenobarbital

    (E) epinephrine

77. The original portion of the Form 222 is eventually kept on file by the

    (A) DEA (B) prescriber (C) FDA

    (D) purchaser (E) supplier

78. A product that contains 60 mg of codeine and 325mg of acetaminophen is most likely to be classified as

    (A) Schedule II (B) Schedule III

    (C) Schedule IV (D) ScheduleV

    (E) Noncontrolled

79. Which of the following are controlled substances?

I. ergotamine tartrate

II. papaverine

III. levorphanol

(A) I only (B) III only (C) I & II only

(D) II & III only (E) I, II, & III

80. Which of the following forms are used to apply for a new DEA registration for a community pharmacy?

I. Form 224

II. Form 222a

III. Form 222

(A) I only (B) III only (C) I & II only

(D) II & III only (E) I, II, & III

81. Which of the following products are Schedule III controlled substances?

I. Tylenol with Codeine #4

II. Fiorinal Capsules

III. Percodan tablets

(A) I only (B) III only (C) I & II only

(D) II & III only (E) I, II, & III

82. Patients treated in an ambulatory care comprehensive narcotic treatment program may receive methadone doses by which of the following routes?

I. IV

II. IM

III. oral

(A) I only (B) III only (C) I & II only

(D) II & III only (E) I, II, & III

83. A new drug product is given the name “felorazepam”. It is likely to be classified as

(A) Schedule II (B) Schedule III
(C) Noncontrolled (D) ScheduleV
(E) Schedule IV

84. An orphan drug is one that has

(A) been removed from the market because of toxicity
(B) has been discontinued because of poor sales
(C) has a low therapeutic index
(D) provided special economic incentives for the manufacturer
(E) has been developed and imported from a foreign country

85. The requirement for over-the-counter drugs to have “adequate directions for use”

(A) means that the directions will be clear to a layperson for safe use of the product.
(B) applies only to products intended for oral consumption
(C) applies only to products for pediatric use
(D) includes the listing of potential side effects and toxicity
(E) includes the presence of bilingual directions

86. Hospital inpatients receiving oral estrogen therapy must receive patient package inserts:

(A) every day
(B) at least every 30 days
(C) only at the first dose and when being discharged
(D) at least every 7 days
(E) only with the first dose

87. Which of the following are Schedule II controlled substances?

   I. morphine tablets
   II. fentanyl injection
   III. tramadol

   (A) I only (B) III only (C) I & II only
   (D) II & III only (E) I, II, & III

88. What permanent identification must a pharmacy possess if it plans to electronically bill Medicare or Medicaid for prescriptions?

   (A) DEA number
   (B) NDC
   (C) FDA registration number
   (D) AWP
   (E) NPI

89. The expiration date on a commercial pharmaceutical product is July 2020. The actual date that this product will be considered expired will be after:

   (A) June 30th (B) July 1st (C) July 15th
   (D) July 31st (E) August 1st

90. A physician who is a resident in a hospital and does not have a DEA registration number

   (A) may not prescribe controlled substances.
   (B) may only prescribe controlled substances for outpatients.
   (C) may prescribe controlled substances using the hospital DEA number plus an assigned suffix.
   (D) may prescribe controlled substances only in Schedule III-V.
   (E) may prescribe only for inpatients.

91. A cosmetic company begins marketing an OTC topical cream that is claimed to reverse psoriatic lesions. This claim may be legally challenged by the:

(A) FDA only (B) HCFA (C) FTC only
(D) DEA (E) FDA and FTC

92. A DEA form 222a is used

(A) to order Schedule II controlled substances
(B) to order all controlled substances
(C) to return unused controlled substances
(D) to order more Form 222 forms
(E) to register a practitioner with DEA

93. Two generic companies manufacture a specific drug in several dosage forms. Which one of the dosage forms is MOST likely to present problems with bioequivalence?

(A) tablet (B) capsule
(C) oral solution (D) parenteral soln.
(E) sustained release tablet

94. Under which of the following situations would a drug product be considered misbranded?

I. An original bottle labeled 50 tablets contains 60 tablets.
II. The concentration of a tetracaine ointment 5 % W/W is only 2%.
III. The manufacturer cannot prove the sterility of a solution labeled "Sterile Diphenhydramine Injection".

(A) I only (B) III only (C) I & II only
(D) II & III only (E) I, II, & III

95. To be admitted to a comprehensive maintenance program, narcotic-dependent individuals must have been physiologically dependent on narcotics for at least

(A) 30 days (B) 90 days (C) 180 days
(D) 12 months (E) 18 months

96. A client requests a refill on a prescription written for Diphenhydramine 25 mg #30 with a Sig reading "one cap 1h before bedtime and 1 hs if needed". There were no indications of refills on the prescription. Which one of the following actions is most appropriate for the pharmacist?

(A) Refuse the refill since no refills were indicated.
(B) Suggest that the client visit a nearby ER for a new prescription.
(C) Give an emergency supply of only 4 capsules.
(D) Advise the purchase of the drug off the shelves since it is an OTC drug.
(E) Suggest that the patient purchase an herbal product for sleep.

97. Which of the following drug products must be purchased by pharmacies using DEA Form 222?

I. Concerta
II. MS Contin
III. Strattera

(A) I only (B) III only (C) I & II only
(D) II & III only (E) I, II, & III

98. Which of the following sublingual tablets do NOT have to be dispensed in child-resistant containers?

I. Isordil
II. Nitrostat
III. Nitroglycerin

(A) I only (B) III only (C) I & II only
(D) II & III only (E) I, II, & III

99. The acronym, DUR, is most closely associated with which of the following?

(A) Drug clinical trials

(B) Medicare reimbursement

(C) Patient counseling

(D) Drug nomenclature

(E) MedWatch

100. Pharmacists are required to periodically inventory supplies of which of the following drug products?

I. Sonata capsules

II. Entex Liquid

III. Sudafed Plus Liquid

(A) I only (B) III only (C) I & II only

(D) II & III only (E) I, II, & III

101. A pharmacist may issue a Power of Attorney to an individual in order to permit the individual to

I. fill controlled substance prescriptions.

II. conduct a narcotic treatment facility.

III. complete DEA Form 222 orders.

(A) I only (B) III only (C) I & II only

(D) II & III only (E) I, II, & III

102. Which of the following drugs are considered to be "Basic Class" drugs under the Controlled Substances Act?

I. dextroamphetamine

II. codeine

III. morphine

(A) I only (B) III only (C) I & II only

(D) II & III only (E) I, II, & III

103. The primary objective or charge for individual state boards of pharmacy is the

(A) enforcement of federal laws

(B) protection of the profession

(C) protection of individual pharmacists

(D) protection of the general public

(E) serving as an intermediary between chain, independent, and institutional pharmacies

104. Under which of the following situations would a drug product be considered adulterated?

I. An herbal product that contains American ginseng rather than the Chinese ginseng listed on the label.

II. A product on the shelf for sale is past its expiration date.

III. A sterile parenteral solution contains a few microorganisms.

(A) I only (B) III only (C) I & II only

(D) II & III only (E) I, II, & III

105. Who is authorized to designate the "official" name for a new drug?

(A) U.S. Congress

(B) Executive Director of APhA

(C) Director of HCFA

(D) Director of the FDA

(E) Secretary of HHS

106. The component of marijuana that is believed to have the most activity to alleviate neuropathic pain, glaucoma and nausea is:

(A) LLB (B) SLM (C) CBD

(D) MLS (E) THC

107. Which of the following was the first to require that pharmaceutical manufacturers prove the safety of prescription drugs before marketing?

(A) Durham-Humphrey Amendment of 1951

(B) Prescription Drug Marketing Act of 1987

(C) Kefauver-Harris Amendment of 1962

(D) F D & C Act of 1938

(E) Pure Food and Drug Act of 1906

108. The advertising to the general public of OTC drugs is basically under the regulatory responsibilities of the:

(A) HCFA (B) FDA and FTC (C) FDA only

(D) DEA (E) FTC only

109. Which dosage forms of secobarbital must be ordered using a DEA Form 222?

I. Suppository

II. Injectable

III. Capsule

(A) I only (B) III only (C) I & II only

(D) II & III only (E) I, II, & III

110. Which portion of the federal counseling regulations must be performed by a committee appointed within each individual state?

I. retrospective review

II. prospective review

III. meta-analysis review

(A) I only (B) III only (C) I & II only

(D) II & III only (E) I, II, & III

111. Which of the following controlled drugs may a pharmacist mail through the US Postal Service?

I. Schedule II's

II. Schedule III's

III. Schedule IV's

(A) I only (B) III only (C) I & II only

(D) II & III only (E) I, II, & III

112. Controlled substance inventories

I. must be made for each registered location.

II. must be taken at least once each year.

III. may be done at any time during the workday.

(A) I only (B) III only (C) I & II only

(D) II & III only (E) I, II, & III

113. Which of the following actions should a pharmacist take if a patient refuses to be counseled about a new prescription?

I. Dispense the prescription but note in the prescription files that counseling was refused.

II. Refuse to dispense the prescription.

III. Dispense the prescription but inform the prescriber that counseling was refused.

(A) I only (B) III only (C) I & II only

(D) II & III only (E) I, II, & III

114. Packaging for nonprescription products that is designed to prevent the addition of foreign material into the final product is best described as being:

(A) tamper-resistant

(B) tamper-evident

(C) tamper-proof

(D) hermetically sealed

(E) air-tight

115. When refilling a prescription that requires a child-resistant container, the pharmacist must always replace which of the following?

I. The plastic closure

II. The plastic container

III. The glass container

(A) I only (B) III only (C) I & II only

(D) II & III only (E) I, II, & III

116. Which of the following is TRUE of Schedule V substances?

I. They all contain codeine.

II. When they are dispensed by the pharmacist, the federal transfer warning must be on the container labeling.

III. Some states may permit sale of these products without a prescription.

(A) I only (B) III only (C) I & II only

(D) II & III only (E) I, II, & III

117. All of the following would be considered as incidences of misbranding EXCEPT

(A) one of the active drug in a product is not identified on the label

(B) the level of alcohol in the product is 5% V/V but the label states 15% V/V

(C) the names of inactive ingredients are not on the label

(D) the original bottle of 60 contains only 50 tablets

(E) the a pharmacist dispenses a drug product without the required prescription authorization

118. In which of the following locations would you NOT find pharmaceutical manufacturer's drug samples?

I. chain or community pharmacy

II. physician's office

III. hospital pharmacy

(A) I only (B) III only (C) I & II only

(D) II & III only (E) I, II, & III

119. Which of the following statements concerning Medicare Plan D is (are) correct?

I. The plan is voluntary for persons on Medicare.

II. Insurance companies may limit prescription drug quantities to 30 day supplies for some drugs.

III. Insurance companies may require participants to receive prescriptions from mail order pharmacies.

(A) I only (B) III only (C) I & II only

(D) II & III only (E) I, II, & III

120. Under which of the following conditions may practitioners of "Traditional Chinese Medicine" sell ephedra-containing products?

(A) The level of ephedra is less than 1 mg per dose.

(B) Only a 10 day supply of product is sold.

(C) A prescription is issued for the product

(D) The label does not indicate that the product is a dietary supplement.

(E) Sales are not legal

121. Which of the following information must be included in the bar code of drug products being sold to hospitals?

I. Expiration dates

II. Lot numbers

III. NDC numbers

(A) I only (B) III only (C) I & II only

(D) II & III only (E) I, II, & III

122. A product that contains not more than 1.8 g of codeine per 100 mL is considered to be in Schedule

(A) I (B) II (C) III
(D) IV (E) V

123. The statement, "Caution: Federal law prohibits the transfer of this drug to any person other than the person for whom it was prescribed" is required on prescription containers for which of the following categories of drugs?

I. Schedule II
II. Schedule III
III. Schedule IV

(A) I only (B) III only (C) I & II only
(D) II & III only (E) I, II, & III

124. Hospitals that plan on using large quantities of tax-free grain alcohol should obtain which one of the following forms?

(A) ATF 1447 (B) ATF 222 (C) DEA 222
(D) ATF 11 (E) DEA 1447

125. Prescriptions for which of the following controlled substances may be partially filled upon request of the patient:

I. Empirin w/codeine #4
II. Subutex
III. Testosterone

(A) I only (B) III only (C) I & II only
(D) II & III only (E) I, II, & III

126. Which of the following is true about DEA Form 222?

I. It may be used by any pharmacy in the same chain
II. It may be partially filled by the supplier
III. A physician may use it to order Schedule II controlled substances

(A) I only (B) III only (C) I & II only
(D) II & III only (E) I, II, & III

127. Dronabinol is a Schedule III controlled substance that is related most closely to

(A) cocaine (B) LSD (C) marijuana
(D) nabumetone (E) methylphenidate

128. Excipients included in pharmaceutical dosage forms are usually listed on which of the following?

(A) DSHEA (B) HPLC (C) GRAS
(D) Top 200 (E) USP

129. Which of the following are examples of Schedule I substances?

I. Lysergic acid diethylamide
II. Mescaline
III. Peyote

(A) I only (B) III only (C) I & II only
(D) II & III only (E) I, II, & III

130. Which of the following actions is (are) permissible under the FDA rules for prescription compounding by pharmacies?

I. Informing an allergist that the pharmacy can economically compound 50 mg diphenhydramine capsules.
II. Sending brochures to nurse practitioners that the pharmacy compounds topical lotions for psoriasis.
III. Advertising to dermatologists that the pharmacy can compound topical antifungal ointments.

(A) I only (B) III only (C) I & II only
(D) II & III only (E) I, II, & III

131. Which of the following is true of DEA Form 222?

I. May be used to transfer Schedule II drugs from one pharmacy to another.

II. May be used to return Schedule II drugs to the supplier.

III. Photocopies of these forms can be used to purchase Schedule II drugs.

(A) I only (B) III only (C) I & II only
(D) II & III only (E) I, II, & III

132. DEA registration numbers that are assigned to mid-level practitioners generally begin with which of the following letters?

(A) M (B) B (C) X
(D) F (E) A

133. The term "Grandfathered" refers to drugs that were marketed before the

(A) DSHEA
(B) Durham-Humphrey Amendment of 1951
(C) FD & C Act of 1938
(D) Kefauver-Harris Amendment of 1962
(E) Poison Prevention Act

134. What number is given to the clinical trial phase that consists of post-marketing surveillance of a drug that was recently introduced onto the market?

(A) 1 (B) 2 (C) 3
(D) 4 (E) 5

135. When conducting a controlled substance inventory, the registrant

   I. must make an exact count of open containers of Schedule II substances.

   II. may estimate the count of a Schedule IV substance in an opened container that originally held 500 tablets.

   III. must make an exact count of all controlled substances in sealed, unopened containers.

   (A) I only (B) III only (C) I & II only

   (D) II & III only (E) I, II, & III

136. Schedule III, IV, and V controlled substance prescriptions may be conveyed to a community pharmacy pursuant to

   I. a fax of a written, signed prescription transmitted by the prescriber to the pharmacy

   II. an oral prescription called in by a prescriber

   III. a written prescription signed by the prescriber

   (A) I only (B) III only (C) I & II only

   (D) II & III only (E) I, II, & III

137. A patient who is being treated with methadone in a narcotic treatment program is admitted to a hospital for the treatment of his pneumonia. How can the client receive his methadone while he is in the hospital?

   I. The patient can be given enough doses at the narcotic treatment program to carry him over his hospital stay.

   II. Authorized nurses can administer methadone to the patient in the hospital in order to maintain or detoxify the patient.

   III. Authorized nurses can administer methadone to the patient in the hospital in order to maintain or detoxify the patient.

   (A) I only (B) III only (C) I & II only

   (D) II & III only (E) I, II, & III

138. Which of the following is/are true regarding the sale of codeine-containing schedule V cough medicine without a prescription?

I. Only a pharmacist may dispense the product to the consumer.

II. A non-pharmacist may "ring-up" the sale and collect payment for the product.

III. Not more than 120 mL or 24 dosage units of this product may be sold to the same purchaser in any 7-day period.

(A) I only (B) III only (C) I & II only
(D) II & III only (E) I, II, & III

139. For which one of the following drugs must a patient sign an informed consent before receiving the original prescription?

(A) olanzapine
(B) morphine sulfate, sustained release
(C) hydrochlorothiazide
(D) almotriptan
(E) tetracycline

140. According to the present DSHEA, an herbal product such as Saw Palmetto may be labeled to state:

(A) cures prostatitis
(B) help treat prostatitis
(C) will return the prostate to normal size
(D) for the prostate
(E) helps in prevention of prostate cancer

141. Which of the following types of products in a hospital pharmacy must be barcoded?

I. prescription drugs

II. biologicals

III. nonprescription drugs

(A) I only (B) III only (C) I & II only

(D) II & III only (E) I, II, & III

142. Pharmacists may transfer prescription information on a one-time basis for the purpose of dispensing a refill for which of the following drug products?

I. Lomotil tablets

II. Dalmane capsules

III. OxyContin

(A) I only (B) III only (C) I & II only

(D) II & III only (E) I, II, & III

143. The names of which of the following ingredients are required to be included on the labels of pharmaceutical products?

I. antimicrobial preservatives

II. coloring agents

III. flavoring oils

(A) I only (B) III only (C) I & II only

(D) II & III only (E) I, II, & III

144. A pharmacist may partially fill a Schedule II prescription

I. and the remaining portion of the prescription may be filled within 72 hours of the partial fill.

II. if the pharmacist does not have enough medication in stock to completely fill the prescription.

III. if the patient only wants some of the medication prescribed.

(A) I only (B) III only (C) I & II only

(D) II & III only (E) I, II, & III

145. A hospital pharmacy director is informed that an employee has been convicted of selling cocaine on the street. Which of the following actions may the director take based upon the Federal Anti-drug Abuse Act of 1988?

I. Warn the employee not to possess or sell illegal drugs in the future.

II. Place a letter of reprimand in the employee's personnel file

III. Terminate the employment of the individual

(A) I only (B) III only (C) I & II only

(D) II & III only (E) I, II, & III

146. A pharmacist receives a prescription for a drug indication that she recognizes as not being a recognized indication for the prescribed drug, but the prescribed use was recently described in the local newspaper. Which of the following actions is most appropriate for the pharmacist?

(A) Fill the prescription.

(B) Fill the prescription but inform the patient that it is not for an appropriate use.

(C) Call the prescriber and inform him that it is illegal to write such a prescription.

(D) Request that the prescriber indicate on the prescription face "off the label use".

(E) Refuse to fill the prescription since is it illegal to fill.

147. A statement that a specific OTC product has a tamper-evident feature may be placed in any of the following locations EXCEPT on the:

(A) closure

(B) tamper-evident device

(C) back of the package

(D) under the product name

(E) front of the package

148. The Drug Quality and Security Act of 2013 is primarily intended to regulate which one of the following entities?

(A) hospitals
(B) foreign drug manufacturers
(C) out-patient clinics
(D) compounding pharmacies
(E) generic manufacturers

149. A prescriber requests information concerning the "off-label" therapeutic use of a drug. In which of the following sources may a pharmacist find such information?

I. TV advertisement sponsored by the drug manufacturer
II. Product Insert
III. AHFS

(A) I only
(B) III only
(C) I & II only
(D) II & III only
(E) I, II, & III

150. Which one of the following must be present on the labels of nonprescription drug products intended for oral use?

(A) Sodium content of active ingredients only
(B) Total sodium content of both active and inactive ingredients
(C) Sodium chloride content of active ingredients
(D) Total sodium chloride content of both active and inactive ingredients
(E) No requirements have been established

151. The *USP/NF* classification system used to describe preparation of HSD's (home-use sterile drug products) uses which of the following terminology?

(A) Low risk versus high risk
(B) Clean rooms 1 through 4
(C) High volume versus low volume
(D) Category A through E
(E) Sterile versus almost sterile

152. A pharmacist observes a misleading prescription drug product advertisement on television. To which one of the following would a complaint be most effective?

(A) APhA
(B) The local Chamber of Commerce
(C) AMA
(D) OPDP
(E) VIPPS

153. According to federal law, a pharmacist must include which of the following on a prescription label?

I. A prescription serial number
II. The name of the manufacturer
III. Expiration date from the manufacturer's label

(A) I only (B) III only (C) I & II only
(D) II & III only (E) I, II, & III

154. Which of the following is (are) true of practitioners who prescribe controlled substances electronically?

I. They may only prescribe Schedule III, IV and V drugs electronically.
II. They may issue prescriptions for up to 3 patients simultaneously with a single signature.
III. They must provide appropriate two-factor authentication credentialing.

(A) I only (B) III only (C) I & II only
(D) II & III only (E) I, II, & III

155. Phenobarbital is a drug that is classified as a(n)

(A) Schedule IV drug
(B) OTC drug
(C) Schedule V drug
(D) non-controlled drug
(E) Schedule III drug

156. For which one of the following drugs must a patient sign an informed consent before receiving an original prescription?

(A) sumatriptan

(B) morphine sulfate, sust. release

(C) paroxetine

(D) isotretinoin

(E) vancomycin

157. Methylphenidate is an example of a drug in controlled substance category

(A) I (B) II (C) III

(D) IV (E) V

158. Which of the following drug products must be purchased using a DEA Form 222?

I. Methadone

II. Amobarbital

III. Fentanyl

(A) I only (B) III only (C) I & II only

(D) II & III only (E) I, II, & III

159. A pharmacist counsels a customer about the purchase of a body lotion which does not contain the coloring agent, tartrazine, to which she is allergic. While examining product labels with the client, the pharmacist should explain that:

I. the concentration of tartrazine present may not be listed.

II. the ingredients, including tartrazine, will be listed alphabetically.

III. rather than list each individual coloring agent, the manufacturer may simply list "yellow dye".

(A) I only (B) III only (C) I & II only

(D) II & III only (E) I, II, & III

160. Orphan drugs are drugs that are
   (A) intended for use in children under the age of 16
   (B) chemically dissimilar to any other marketed drug moiety
   (C) used in the treatment of rare diseases
   (D) intended for use in children under the age of 5
   (E) administered to children without the permission of their parents

161. The purchasing agent of your hospital suggests that the hospital purchase a two-year supply of a popular antibiotic at a special price. Which of the following are legal activities?
   I. sell a portion of the antibiotic to a community pharmacy
   II. sell a portion of the antibiotic to another area hospital
   III. purchase of that quantity of the antibiotic
   (A) I only (B) III only (C) I & II only
   (D) II & III only (E) I, II, & III

162. Drug products with which of the following codes may be substituted for one another?
   I. B
   II. AB
   III. A
   (A) I only (B) III only (C) I & II only
   (D) II & III only (E) I, II, & III

163. The major objective of the Electronic Orange Book is to compare drug products that are
   I. multisourced
   II. most economical
   III. different dosage forms
   (A) I only (B) III only (C) I & II only
   (D) II & III only (E) I, II, & III

164. Which of the following are permissible when taking a controlled substance inventory?

I. assistance of a technician to count tablets

II. use of a recording device

III. maintaining inventory records on a recording device

(A) I only (B) III only (C) I & II only

(D) II & III only (E) I, II, & III

165. Under which one of the following Acts are biological products classified as "biosimilars"?

(A) Durham-Humphrey Amendment

(B) Health Care Act

(C) FDA Modernization Act

(D) Prescription Drug Marketing

(E) Orphan Drug

166. A 35-year old customer wishes to know how many 30 mg Sudafed tablets he can purchase at one time. Which of the following is the correct answer?

(A) 12 (B) 60 (C) 120

(D) 240 (E) 300

167. While presenting a talk on drug abuse, a pharmacist is asked for information concerning the "date-rape drugs". Her response may include which of the following?

I. These drugs are Schedule II substances.

II. The generic name for the drug is gamma-hydroxybutyric acid.

III. The therapeutic classification of one of these drugs is as a behavioral depressant and hypnotic.

(A) I only (B) III only (C) I & II only

(D) II & III only (E) I, II, & III

168. Which of the following protocols must a hospital pharmacy follow in order to possess pharmaceutical manufacturer's drug samples?

I. The hospital must be registered as a drug wholesaler.

II. A licensed practitioner must have requested the samples from the company.

III. The hospital must store the samples separate from the regular stock.

(A) I only (B) III only (C) I & II only
(D) II & III only (E) I, II, & III

169. What is the time interval during which newly eligible individuals may enroll in Medicare Plan D without a penalty?

(A) 3 months (B) 6 months (C) 7 months
(D) 9 months (E) 1 year

170. Which of the following items must be ordered from a wholesaler on DEA order form 222?

I. Percocet

II. ketamine 50mg/mL

III. diazepam tablets 10 mg

(A) I only (B) III only (C) I & II only
(D) II & III only (E) I, II, & III

171. Which of the following is NOT required on the label of unit dose packages prepared in a hospital?

(A) name of the drug
(B) manufacturer's expiration date
(C) control number
(D) strength of drug
(E) beyond-use expiration dating

172. Which of the following volumes of the USP DI contains significant information concerning the bioequivalence of drug products?

I. Volume I

II. Volume II

III. Volume III

(A) I only (B) III only (C) I & II only
(D) II & III only (E) I, II, & III

173. Which of the following statements concerning drug recalls is (are) accurate?

I. They occur only after fatalities have occurred.

II. They may be ordered by the FDA.

III. They may be voluntary actions by the pharmaceutical manufacturer.

(A) I only (B) III only (C) I & II only
(D) II & III only (E) I, II, & III

174. The term used in the HIPAA privacy rules to describe the removal of patient identifying information when discussing a specific clinical case in public is:

(A) depersonalization

(B) debriefing

(C) document erasure

(D) de-indentification

(E) anti-terrorist protection

175. A faxed Schedule II prescription from the prescriber to a pharmacy is permitted

I. if the patient is a hospice patient..

II. if the patient is a resident of a LTCF

III. at any time as long as it is followed by a written "cover" prescription.

(A) I only (B) III only (C) I & II only
(D II & III only (E) I, II, & III

176. Uses for tax-free alcohol purchased by a hospital may include:

I. incorporation into formulas for inpatient orders.

II. incorporation into prescriptions for outpatients.

III. selling of small amounts to independent pharmacies based upon their immediate prescription needs.

(A) I only (B) III only (C) I & II only
(D) II & III only (E) I, II, & III

177. Which of the following categories of drugs require the legend "Rx only" to be on the manufacturer's package?

I. Schedule V controlled drugs

II. Schedule II controlled drugs

III. Schedule III and IV controlled drugs

(A) I only (B) III only (C) I & II only
(D) II & III only (E) I, II, & III

178. The iPLEDGE program is intended to assure appropriate and safe dispensing of which one of the following drugs?

(A) cyclosporine (B) sildenafil (C) nevirapine
(D) thalidomide (E) isotretinoin

179. The first series of digits in the NDC for a drug product represents the:

(A) drug name (B) drug strength
(C) package size (D) therapeutic use
(E) manufacturer

Figure A

TE Code	RLD	Active Ingredient	Dosage Form; Route	Strength	Proprietary Name	Applicant
AB	No	WARFARIN	TABLET; ORAL	1MG	COUMADIN	BRISTOL MYERS SQUIBB (BMS)
AB	No	WARFARIN	TABLET; ORAL	2MG	COUMADIN	BMS
AB	No	WARFARIN	TABLET; ORAL	5MG	COUMADIN	BMS
AB	Yes	WARFARIN	TABLET; ORAL	10MG	COUMADIN	BMS
AB	No	WARFARIN	TABLET; ORAL	2MG	WARFARIN	BARR
AB	No	WARFARIN	TABLET; ORAL	5MG	WARFARIN	BARR
AB	No	WARFARIN	TABLET; ORAL	10MG	WARFARIN	BARR
AB	No	WARFARIN	TABLET; ORAL	2MG	WARFARIN	INVAMED
AB	No	WARFARIN	TABLET; ORAL	5MG	WARFARIN	INVAMED
AB	No	WARFARIN	TABLET; ORAL	10MG	WARFARIN	INVAMED

180. A prescription is written for Coumadin tablets 5 mg with an indication that substitution is desired. Which of the following manufacturers have suitable products? (see Figure A).

I. Bristol Myers Squibb
II. Invamed
III. Barr

(A) I only (B) III only (C) I & II only
(D) II & III only (E) I, II, & III

181. A prescription is written for warfarin tablets 2 mg with an indication that substitution is desired. Which of the following manufacturers have suitable products? (See Figure A)

I. Bristol Myers Squibb (BMS)
II. Invamed
III. Barr

(A) I only (B) III only (C) I & II only
(D) II & III only (E) I, II, & III

182. In order to be considered bioequivalent with Bristol Myers Squibb's Coumadin tablets, Barr's warfarin sodium tablets must have about the same (See Figure A):

I. color

II. excipients

III. AUC

(A) I only (B) III only (C) I & II only

(D) II & III only (E) I, II, & III

183. Partial filling of a schedule IV controlled substance prescription is permissible, provided that

I. each partial filling is recorded.

II. the total quantity dispensed in all partial fillings does not exceed the total quantity prescribed.

III. the total price charged for the partial fillings does not exceed the total price the patient would have paid with a complete filling of the prescription.

(A) I only (B) III only (C) I & II only

(D) II & III only (E) I, II, & III

184. Which of the following is true about DEA Form 222?

I. If any forms are lost, the loss must be reported to DEA.

II. If an order cannot be filled by a supplier the form must be returned to the purchaser.

III. If it contains incorrect information the supplier may correct it and initial the correction.

(A) I only (B) III only (C) I & II only

(D) II & III only (E) I, II, & III

185. An inspector from the FDA enters your community pharmacy. He/she may issue citations if which of the following are found?

I. Drug samples being sold /dispensed pursuant to a prescription.

II. Recalled prescription drugs among the drug stock.

III. Samples stored in the drug stock.

(A) I only (B) III only (C) I & II only
(D) II & III only (E) I, II, & III

186. Davis Labs is the first to place a new drug entity on the market. This product would be described in the Electronic Orange Book as:

I. AB rated.

II. B rated.

III. a reference drug product.

(A) I only (B) III only (C) I & II only
(D) II & III only (E) I, II, & III

187. Ephedra may no longer be present in which of the following products in a community pharmacy?

I. Nonprescription drug products

II. Herbal teas

III. Dietary supplements

(A) I only (B) III only (C) I & II only
(D) II & III only (E) I, II, & III

188. The pharmacist manager of a community pharmacy enters the pharmacy and finds that a variety of controlled products have been stolen over night. Which of the following is required to do?

(A) Complete and send to DEA the Form 204

(B) Lock the pharmacy area until a DEA agent has examined the site.

(C) Complete and send to DEA the Form 106

(D) Contact the board of pharmacy before the pharmacy is open.

(E) Complete and send to DEA the Form 184a

189. Which of the following drug products are exempt from the requirements of the Poison Prevention Packaging Act?

I. Nitroglycerin SL tablets

II. Potassium supplements in unit dose packets

III. Tablets used for erectile dysfunction

(A) I only (B) III only (C) I & II only

(D) II & III only (E) I, II, & III

190. Schedule II prescriptions

I. may only be refilled once.

II. may be partially filled under certain conditions.

III. written for a hospice patient may be faxed to a pharmacy.

(A) I only (B) III only (C) I & II only

(D) II & III only (E) I, II, & III

191. What acronym is used by the USP to designate sterile products that are prepared in a home infusion pharmacy for delivery to a patient's home residence?

(A) SP (B) LVP (C) PPI

(D) HSD (E) TRP

192. The federal act that specifically limits the re-importation of drug products that were previously exported by a pharmaceutical manufacturer is the:

(A) Prescription Drug Marketing Act of 1987
(B) Durham-Humphrey Amendment of 1951
(C) FD & C Act of 1938
(D) DSHEA
(E) Kefauver-Harris Amendment of 1962

193. Which of the following is NOT considered to be a Mid-Level Practitioner?

(A) Dental Assistant (B) Nurse Midwife
(C) Optometrist (D) Veterinarian
(E) Nurse Anesthetist

194. Zolpidem is an example of a drug product in controlled substance schedule

(A) I (B) II (C) III
(D) IV (E) V

195. Which of the following statements is (are) true with respect to the National Drug Code (NDC)?

I. NDC must be imprinted on tablets.
II. NDC must be imprinted on capsules.
III. Every prescription drug product marketed in the US must have an NDC.

(A) I only (B) III only (C) I & II only
(D) II & III only (E) I, II, & III

196. Short-term narcotic detoxification is defined as treatment that is for a period of less than

(A) 90 days (B) 60 days (C) 30 days
(D) 180 days (E) 1 year

197. Which one of the following types of information is useful but not mandatory on the labels of OTC products?

(A) name of manufacturer (B) address of manufacturer
(C) net contents (D) adequate directions for use
(E) NDC number

198. Which of the following drug products is/are NOT classified as a controlled substance?

I. Toviaz
II. Ramelteon
III. Actiq

(A) I only (B) III only (C) I & II only
(D) II & III only (E) I, II, & III

199. Which of the following are Schedule I controlled substances?

I. lysergic acid diethylamide
II. mescaline
III. methaqualone

(A) I only (B) III only (C) I & II only
(D) II & III only (E) I, II, & III

200. Which of the following is TRUE?

I. Original schedule III, IV, or V prescriptions may be transferred from one pharmacy to another for the purpose of refill dispensing.
II. Information from schedule III, IV, or V prescriptions may not be transferred to another pharmacy unless authorized by the prescriber to do so.
III. Pharmacies electronically sharing a real-time, online database may transfer refills to one another as long as the number of refills transferred does not exceed those authorized by the prescriber or the law.

(A) I only (B) III only (C) I & II only
(D) II & III only (E) I, II, & III

201. Which of the following are Schedule II controlled substances?

I. sufentanil

II. propofol

III. midazolam

(A) I only (B) III only (C) I & II only

(D) II & III only (E) I, II, & III

202. Therapeutic substitution is allowed only if an institution is:

(A) nonprofit

(B) for profit

(C) licensed to do so

(D) using a formulary system

(E) under the supervision of a Pharm.D. graduate

203. The statement "Rx only" must appear on which of the following types of drug products

I. orphan drugs

II. controlled substance drugs

III. pediatric drugs

(A) I only (B) III only (C) I & II only

(D) II & III only (E) I, II, & III

204. Which organization is primarily responsible for evaluating the safety and effectiveness of drugs used in veterinary practices?

(A) SPCA (B) FTC (C) FDA

(D) VIPP (E) HCFA

205. Which one of the following designations for drug products that require a prescription in the United States has replaced the designation "Caution: Federal law prohibits dispensing without a prescription"?

(A) Do not dispense without a prescription.
(B) Rx only
(C) Federal law prohibits use by anyone other than the original patient.
(D) Legend drug
(E) Do not transfer to a third party.

206. Patients that attempt to purchase drugs from online websites should look for the following medallion on the website.

(A) APhA
(B) Good Housekeeping Approval
(C) NARD
(D) VIPPS
(E) USAN

207. The *USP/NF* is best described as a publication that is published by:

(A) the HHS
(B) the FDA
(C) the Pharmaceutical Manufacturer's Association
(D) USP Pharmacopeial Convention
(E) a coalition of US pharmaceutical companies

208. With respect to pregnancy warnings, category D indicates that the drug

(A) is safe for 98% of all females during pregnancy.
(B) should not be used during the first trimester.
(C) should be administered only if the potential benefits are acceptable despite the potential risks.
(D) should not be used during pregnancy.
(E) does not pose any danger to either the mother or fetus.

209. Which one of the following is MOST important to consider in determining whether a community pharmacy is required to meet HIPAA regulations?

(A) The prescription volume is greater than 20,000 per year.

(B) Identifiable patient health information is transferred electronically.

(C) The pharmacy accepts Medicaid prescriptions.

(D) The store's annual income is greater than one million dollars.

(E) The pharmacy has more than 10 employees.

210. Which of the following is true?

I. Prescribers must keep records of all controlled substances that they dispense directly to the patient.

II. Prescribers must keep records of all controlled substances administered in the course of narcotic detoxification treatment.

III. Prescribers must keep records of all controlled substances that they receive as samples.

(A) I only (B) III only (C) I & II only

(D) II & III only (E) I, II, & III

211. Which of the following are NOT true of electronic prescribing of controlled substances?

I. Only Pharm. D. graduates may fill an electronic prescription for a controlled substance.

II. After prescribing an electronic controlled substance prescription, it must be followed-up by a written prescription within 72 hours.

III. All prescriptions must be prescribed electronically by 2016.

(A) I only (B) III only (C) I & II only

(D) II & III only (E) I, II, & III

212. When a patient begins a comprehensive narcotic treatment program, the first day's dose of methadone must generally not exceed

(A) 0.5 mg (B) 1 mg (C) 5 mg
(D) 20 mg (E) 40 mg

213. A new cough syrup contains 15 mg of codeine phosphate and 100 mg of guaifenesin in each 10 mL dose. A 4 fluid ounce container of this product would likely be classified as

(A) Schedule II
(B) Schedule III
(C) Schedule IV
(D) Schedule V
(E) Noncontrolled

214. Narcotic drugs may be dispensed to treat narcotic dependence in which of the following facilities?

I. Any institutional pharmacy
II. Any facility with a DEA certified narcotic treatment counselor
III. FDA and state approved narcotic treatment programs

(A) I only (B) III only (C) I & II only
(D) II & III only (E) I, II, & III

215. When a pharmacist conducts a controlled substance inventory, which of the following must be included?

I. Drugs stored in a warehouse for the registrant at a different location.
II. Drugs ordered by a customer but not yet paid for.
III. All controlled substances dispensed over the past 30 days.

(A) I only (B) III only (C) I & II only
(D) II & III only (E) I, II, & III

216. A hospital that has two 55-gallon drums of tax-free grain alcohol must:
   (A) maintain a running inventory of the volume
   (B) inventory the stock every month
   (C) inventory the stock every 6 months
   (D) report the amount remaining to the ATF every six months
   (E) take a year-end inventory

217. Which form must a community pharmacy use to purchase grain alcohol for compounding purposes?
   (A) FDA 23a (B) ATF 1447 (C) DEA 222
   (D) DEA 23a (E) ATF 11

218. A pharmacist may refuse to accept or fill a prescription under all of the following circumstances EXCEPT when:
   (A) the prescription is suspected to be either forged or fictitiously written.
   (B) the pharmacist believes that the drug product may be harmful to the patient.
   (C) the pharmacist believes that he will be violating the law by filling the prescription.
   (D) the patient is known to be HIV positive.
   (E) the drug or drug product is not in stock.

219. Any physician is permitted to
   I. administer drugs to relieve acute narcotic withdrawal symptoms.
   II. prescribe drugs to relieve acute narcotic withdrawal symptoms.
   III. administer drugs to provide narcotic drug-dependent patients with maintenance treatment.
   (A) I only (B) III only (C) I & II only
   (D) II & III only (E) I, II, & III

220. Samples of prescription drugs received from pharmaceutical companies may be
   (A) given to patients by a prescriber.
   (B) dispensed from a hospital pharmacy for inpatients.
   (C) dispensed from a hospital to outpatients.
   (D) sold through community pharmacies.
   (E) traded to another pharmacy for other drugs.

221. Which of the following was the first to require that pharmaceutical manufacturers prove the efficacy of prescription drugs before marketing?
   (A) Prescription Drug Marketing Act of 1987
   (B) FD & C Act of 1938
   (C) Durham-Humphrey Amendment of 1951
   (D) Kefauver-Harris Amendment of 1962
   (E) Pure Food and Drug Act of 1906

222. Which of the following categories of pregnancy warnings is the most severe?
   (A) Category A (B) Category D
   (C) Category III (D) Category X
   (E) Category NR

223. Copy 3 of DEA Form 222 is eventually kept by the
   (A) FDA (B) supplier (C) DEA
   (D) prescriber (E) purchaser

224. Which of the drug products used to treat narcotic dependence is (are) available in a sublingual dosage form?
   I. Methadone
   II. Subutex
   III. Suboxone
   (A) I only (B) III only (C) I & II only
   (D) II & III only (E) I, II, & III

225. The label of a bottle of Ipecac Syrup sold OTC for accidental poisoning must:

I. have its warnings printed in red ink.

II. contain the telephone number of the regional poison control center.

III. state that the appropriate dose is the entire bottle followed by a full glass of water.

(A) I only (B) III only (C) I & II only
(D) II & III only (E) I, II, & III

226. The code, shape and color that is imprinted on each commercial oral tablet must provide which of the following information?

I. manufacturer or distributor

II. name and strength of the drug

III. date of manufacturing

(A) I only (B) III only (C) I & II only
(D) II & III only (E) I, II, & III

227. "Tall Man Lettering" is used to

(A) calculate a drug dose using height

(B) calculate a drug dose using height and weight

(C) print prescription labels for the visually handicapped

(D) print labels for solutions to be administered by IV infusion

(E) reduce medication errors

228. A pharmacy has been compounding a psoriasis cream in 30-gram jars based upon prescriptions written by physicians in a local dermatology clinic. Under which of the following circumstances could the pharmacy also dispense the jars?

I. For patients of other prescribers based upon written prescriptions

II. To the original dermatology clinic for dispensing by the dermatologists

III. To other pharmacies provided they provide a written purchase order

(A) I only (B) III only (C) I & II only
(D) II & III only (E) I, II, & III

229. A pharmaceutical company requests the names and addresses of patients who have received a certain antidepressant drug during the past month.

I. The request may be honored if the company gives the pharmacist an affidavit that a list of the patients' names and addresses will not leave the company.

II. The request is appropriate if the company only wishes to send the patients information concerning depression.

III. Honoring this request will represent a breach of privacy based upon the Federal Health Insurance Portability and Accountability Act.

(A) I only (B) III only (C) I & II only
(D) II & III only (E) I, II, & III

230. Which of the following apply to prescriptions for isotretinoin?

   I. Not more than a one month supply may be dispensed.
   II. The prescription must be filled within 30 days of issue.
   III. Not more than 3 refills may be authorized on the original prescription.

   (A) I only (B) III only (C) I & II only
   (D) II & III only (E) I, II, & III

231. Which of the following designations indicate that drug products of the same strength and dosage form may be interchangeable?

   I. A
   II. AB
   III. BC

   (A) I only (B) III only (C) I & II only
   (D) II & III only (E) I, II, & III

232. Which of the following employees may administer or dispense drugs to patients as part of a narcotic treatment program?

   I. Pharmacists
   II. Registered nurses
   III. Licensed practical nurses

   (A) I only (B) III only (C) I & II only
   (D) II & III only (E) I, II, & III

233. Every new drug placed on the market will have a designated

   I. trade name
   II. brand name
   III. generic name

   (A) I only (B) III only (C) I & II only
   (D) II & III only (E) I, II, & III

234. A drug product consisting of tablets may be declared misbranded under all of the following guidelines EXCEPT:

(A) portion of the label is misleading

(B) label does not indicate number of tablets present

(C) official names of certain ingredients not used

(D) name and location of manufacturer is missing

(E) tablets do not meet assay limits

235. Who must be registered with the DEA in order for a hospital pharmacy to dispense controlled substances?

I. The hospital pharmacy

II. The chief pharmacist

III. Every pharmacist who dispenses on a regular basis

(A) I only (B) III only (C) I & II only

(D) II & III only (E) I, II, & III

236. Oral orders for Schedule II drugs may be accepted and dispensed by a pharmacist

I. if a patient is a regular customer of the pharmacy.

II. if the physician is more than 100 miles away from the pharmacy.

III. in an emergency situation.

(A) I only (B) III only (C) I & II only

(D) II & III only (E) I, II, & III

237. Which of the following drug products are controlled substances?

I. Risperdal

II. Ativan

III. Lyrica

(A) I only (B) III only (C) I & II only

(D) II & III only (E) I, II, & III

238. Major objectives for developing a formulary include:

I. give prescribers a greater latitude of drug selection

II. allow therapeutic substitution

III. reduce drug inventory

(A) I only (B) III only (C) I & II only

(D) II & III only (E) I, II, & III

239. Which of the following populations are covered under the Medicare Modernization Act of 2003?

I. Medicare beneficiaries

II. Nongovernmental employees

III. Medicaid beneficiaries

(A) I only (B) III only (C) I & II only

(D) II & III only (E) I, II, & III

240. A community pharmacy develops and prepares batches of 5,000 sustained release capsules similar to a commercially available product but at a lower price. The pharmacy may be cited for this activity based upon:

I. The formula may be considered a new drug

II. The failure to following GMPs.

III. The preparation of 5,000 capsules may be considered manufacturing.

(A) I only (B) III only (C) I & II only

(D) II & III only (E) I, II, & III

241. A prescription calls for Nitro-Dur transdermal patch 0.1 mg/hr. Which of the following transdermal products may be dispensed if substitution is required? (See Figures B & C)

I. Novartis's NTG 0.1 mg/hr.

II. Mylan's NTG 0.1 mg/hr.

III. 3M's Minitran 0.1 mg/hr.

(A) I only (B) III only (C) I & II only

(D) II & III only (E) I, II, & III

Figure B

TE Code	RLD	Active Ingredient	Dosage Form; Route	Strength	Proprietary Name	Applicant
AB1	Yes	NITRO-GLYCERIN	Film, Extended Release; Transdermal	0.1 MG/HR	NITRO-DUR	KEY
AB1	Yes	NITRO-GLYCERIN	"	0.2 MG/HR	NITRO-DUR	KEY
AB1	Yes	NITRO-GLYCERIN	"	0.4 MG/HR	NITRO-DUR	KEY
AB1	Yes	NITRO-GLYCERIN	"	0.6 MG/HR	NITRO-DUR	KEY
AB1	Yes	NITRO-GLYCERIN	"	0.8 MG/HR	NITRO-DUR	KEY
AB1	No	NITRO-GLYCERIN	Film, Extended Release; Transdermal	0.1 MG/HR	MINITRAN	3M
AB1	No	NITRO-GLYCERIN	"	0.2 MG/HR	MINITRAN	3M
AB1	No	NITRO-GLYCERIN	"	0.4 MG/HR	MINITRAN	3M
AB1	No	NITRO-GLYCERIN	"	0.6 MG/HR	MINITRAN	3M

242. Which of the following companies' 0.2 mg/hr nitroglycerin patches are considered to be interchangeable when substituting? (See Figures B & C)

I. Hercon Labs

II. Mylan

III. Novartis

(A) I only (B) III only (C) I & II only

(D) II & III only (E) I, II, & III

Figure C

TE Code	RLD	Active Ingredient	Dosage Form; Route	Strength	Proprietary Name	Applicant
AB2	Yes	NITRO-GLYCERIN	Film, Extended Release; Transdermal	0.1 MG/HR	TRANS-DERM-NITRO	NOVARTIS
AB2	Yes	NITRO-GLYCERIN		0.2 MG/HR	TRANS-DERM-NITRO	NOVARTIS
AB2	Yes	NITRO-GLYCERIN		0.4 MG/HR	TRANS-DERM-NITRO	NOVARTIS
AB2	Yes	NITRO-GLYCERIN		0.6 MG/HR	TRANS-DERM-NITRO	NOVARTIS
AB2	No	NITRO-GLYCERIN		0.2 MG/HR	NITRO-GLYCERIN	HERCON
AB2	No	NITRO-GLYCERIN		0.4 MG/HR	NITRO-GLYCERIN	HERCON
AB2	No	NITRO-GLYCERIN		0.6 MG/HR	NITRO-GLYCERIN	HERCON
AB2	No	NITRO-GLYCERIN		0.1 MG/HR	NITRO-GLYCERIN	MYLAN
AB2	No	NITRO-GLYCERIN		0.2 MG/HR	NITRO-GLYCERIN	MYLAN
AB2	No	NITRO-GLYCERIN		0.4 MG/HR	NITRO-GLYCERIN	MYLAN
AB2	No	NITRO-GLYCERIN		0.6 MG/HR	NITRO-GLYCERIN	MYLAN
AP	Yes	NITRO-GLYCERIN	Injectable; Injection	5 MG/mL	NITRO-GLYCERIN	ABBOTT
AP	Yes	NITRO-GLYCERIN	Injectable; Injection	5 MG/mL	NITRO-GLYCERIN	NOVARTIS

243. A prescription order is written "NTG injection 5 mg/mL". Which of the following statements is (are) true based upon Figure C?

    I. Abbott's product may be used.

    II. Nitroglycerin injection by Novartis may be used.

    III. The AP classification indicates that the products are

interchangeable.

(A) I only (B) III only (C) I & II only
(D) II & III only (E) I, II, & III

244. A prescription order is written "NTG transdermal patch 0.4 mg/hr. Do NOT substitute. Which of the following companies' product(s) could the pharmacist dispense? (See Figure C)

I. Novartis
II. Hercon
III. Mylan

(A) I only (B) III only (C) I & II only
(D) II & III only (E) I, II, & III

245. A prescription order is written "Tranderm-Nitro 0.4 mg/hr". Assuming that substitution is NOT permissible, which of the following companies' products could be used? (See Figure C)

I. Novartis
II. Mylan
III. Hercon

(A) I only (B) III only (C) I & II only
(D) II & III only (E) I, II, & III

246. A pharmacy carries a complete stock of Nitro-Dur and Minitran patches. In which of the following strengths are these two lines considered bioequivalent? (See Figure B)

I. 0.2 mg/hr
II. 0.4 mg/hr
III. 0.6 mg/hr

(A) I only (B) III only (C) I & II only
(D) II & III only (E) I, II, & III

247. Labels on cosmetic packages must have ingredients listed:

(A) in ascending order of concentration.

(B) with the most active listed first.

(C) alphabetically.

(D) any random order.

(E) in descending order of concentration.

248. A pharmacy that compounds large numbers of prescriptions may be cited by the FDA if its volume of prescriptions being sent to out-of-state is in excess of ____ %.

(A) 5 (B) 75 (C) 40

(D) 10 (E) 25

249. Which of the products listed below would be considered to be Schedule III controlled substances?

I. A product that contains 90 mg of codeine per dose.

II. A product that contains 15 mg of hydrocodone per dose.

III. A product that contains 2.5 mg of diphenoxylate and 25 mcg of atropine sulfate per dose.

(A) I only (B) III only (C) I & II only

(D) II & III only (E) I, II, & III

250. Which of the following products is (are) approved for the treatment of narcotic dependence?

I. Methadone

II. Subutex

III. Buspirone

(A) I only (B) III only (C) I & II only

(D) II & III only (E) I, II, & III

251. Based upon federal law, which of the following schedules of controlled substances may be dispersed throughout the prescription drug stock of a community pharmacy?

I. Schedule II's

II. Schedule III's

III. Schedule IV and V's

(A) I only (B) III only (C) I & II only

(D) II & III only (E) I, II, & III

252. The statement "Caution: Federal law prohibits the transfer of this drug to any person other than the patient for whom it was prescribed" is NOT required for

I. controlled substances dispensed for use in "blinded" clinical investigations.

II. dispensing Schedule V drugs.

III. dispensing controlled substances to be administered to a patient in an institution.

(A) I only (B) III only (C) I & II only

(D) II & III only (E) I, II, & III

253. Which of the following statements on a cranberry extract label would be acceptable under DSHEA regulations?

I. To reduce E coli counts during a UTI.

II. To reduce the incidence and duration of UTI's.

III. To help maintain a healthy urinary tract in females.

(A) I only (B) III only (C) I & II only

(D) II & III only (E) I, II, & III

254. A pharmaceutical manufacturer requests from a community pharmacy the names and addresses of patients receiving the company's antidepressant so that a special discount coupons may be provided for future prescriptions. This scenario is probably in violation of which of the following laws?

(A) HIPAA
(B) FDA Modernization Act of 1997
(C) OBRA 90
(D) DSHEA
(E) Sherman Antitrust Act

255. If a specific lot of a pharmaceutical company's tablets fails to meet the expected expiration dating, the lot may be considered to be:

(A) adulterated (B) unstable (C) misbranded
(D) a class III recall (E) a felony

256. In the United States the name designated on the label of an herbal product must conform to that listed in which one of the following reference sources?

(A) Herbal Medicine (German Commission E)
(B) Tyler's Popular Herbs
(C) Physicians' Desk Reference
(D) Remington – The Science and Practice of Pharmacy
(E) AHPA's Herbs of Commerce

257. The classification of drugs into controlled substance schedules by the federal government is based upon the drug's

I. potential for abuse and dependence
II. therapeutic index
III. toxicity

(A) I only (B) III only (C) I & II only
(D) II & III only (E) I, II, & III

258. Which of the following is a characteristic of narrow therapeutic index drugs?
   (A) Large differences between median lethal dose and median effective dose.
   (B) Large differences between minimum toxic concentration and minimum effective concentration.
   (C) Small differences between therapeutic and toxic doses.
   (D) Not more than a 30 days' supply may be dispensed to a patient at one time.
   (E) Patients are required to have regular blood tests performed.

259. Which one of the following laws first required the statement "Caution: Federal law prohibits dispensing without a prescription" on drug product packaging?
   (A) FD & C Act of 1938
   (B) Durham-Humphrey Amendment of 1951
   (C) Kefauver-Harris Amendment
   (D) Prescription Drug Marketing Act
   (E) Pure Food and Drug Act of 1906

260. Which of the following are Schedule IV controlled substances?
   I. chlordiazepoxide
   II. halazepam
   III. nandrolone
   (A) I only (B) III only (C) I & II only
   (D) II & III only (E) I, II, & III

261. Which of the following barbiturates is classified in controlled substance category IV?

I. Phenobarbital

II. Pentobarbital

III. Amobarbital

(A) I only (B) III only (C) I & II only

(D) II & III only (E) I, II, & III

262. Which of the following is true of DEA Form 222?

I. It is used to order Schedule II controlled substances.

II. Only one product may be ordered on each line of the form.

III. May be used to order syringes and hypodermic needles.

(A) I only (B) III only (C) I & II only

(D) II & III only (E) I, II, & III

263. Which of the following products are exempt from the FDA regulations concerning expiration dating?

I. *USP/NF* drug products

II. dietary supplements

III. vitamins

(A) I only (B) III only (C) I & II only

(D) II & III only (E) I, II, & III

264. Which one of the following actions is permissible in a hospital that has tax-free alcohol?

(A) sell pint quantities to physician offices

(B) loan pint quantities to community pharmacies

(C) dispensing to inpatients in the form of a tonic

(D) sell pint quantities to community pharmacies

(E) loan pint quantities to other hospitals

265. Which of the following are Schedule IV controlled substances?

I. zaleplon
II. buprenorphine
III. methylphenidate

(A) I only (B) III only (C) I & II only
(D) II & III only (E) I, II, & III

266. Which one of the following dosage forms is LEAST likely to present bioequivalence problems?

(A) capsule
(B) tablet
(C) IV solution
(D) transdermal patch
(E) suspension

267. Sponsors of Medicare Plan D programs must provide a broad choice of formulary drugs for each of the following drug categories EXCEPT:

(A) anticonvulsants
(B) antidepressants
(C) antihyperlipidemics
(D) antineoplastics
(E) antipsychotics

268. A filled DEA Form 222 must be kept by the

I. DEA for 10 years
II. purchaser for 3 years
III. supplier for 2 years

(A) I only (B) III only (C) I & II only
(D) II & III only (E) I, II, & III

269. In the U.S., which of the following commercial drug products intended for oral administration must have an identifying imprint on each individual dosage unit?

I. Nonprescription tablets

II. Prescription tablets

III. Prescription capsules

(A) I only (B) III only (C) I & II only

(D) II & III only (E) I, II, & III

270. Which one of the following acronyms is most closely associated with health care reimbursement?

(A) DEA (B) DRG (C) GMP

(D) JCAHO (E) PPI

271. Blood and/or urine tests are frequently performed on participants in comprehensive narcotic maintenance treatment programs in order to detect

I. continued abuse of drugs

II. hepatotoxicity

III. drug toxicity

(A) I only (B) III only (C) I & II only

(D) II & III only (E) I, II, & III

272. Evidence indicates that a marketed drug product may have a new use for another condition. In order to claim this new indication, a drug manufacturer must:

(A) submit an abbreviated NDA

(B) apply for patent protection

(C) submit a NDA

(D) submit a supplemental NDA

(E) inform FDA in writing of the revised labeling

273. How may a physician obtain cocaine HCl powder for use as a local anesthetic in his office?

I. By ordering it directly from a supplier using DEA Form 222.

II. By writing an order for the drug in an institutional setting and writing "for office use" on its face

III. By writing a prescription for the drug and writing "for office use" on its face.

(A) I only (B) III only (C) I & II only
(D) II & III only (E) I, II, & III

274. How often must a pharmacy have a patient sign a new notice that he/she has been informed of the pharmacy's privacy practices under HIPAA requirements?

(A) Every time a new prescription is filled
(B) Every time a refill is dispensed
(C) Every 6 months
(D) Every year
(E) No requirements are specified by HIPAA

275. The Consumer Product Safety Commission is responsible for which one of the following?

(A) Federal Food, Drug and Cosmetic Act
(B) Poison Prevention Packaging Act
(C) Prescription drug to OTC status
(D) Good Manufacturing Practice program
(E) DSHEA

276. What is the longest "beyond use" expiration date that a pharmacist may place on a prescription container if the original drug container label states "expiration date 1/2020"? Assume the pharmacist fills the prescription on January 2, 2017.

(A) 7/2/17 (B) 1/2/18 (C) 7/2/18
(D) 1/1/20 (E) 1/31/20

277. A customer enters your pharmacy and requests 25 quinine 260 mg tablets. Which of the following responses by the pharmacist would be appropriate?

I. Quinine tablets can no longer be sold over-the-counter.

II. OTC quinine is considered to be unsafe for the prevention of malaria.

III. OTC quinine is considered ineffective for the treatment of nocturnal leg cramps.

(A) I only (B) III only (C) I & II only
(D) II & III only (E) I, II, & III

278. According to Federal regulations, a color additive may not be added to which one of the following dosage forms?

(A) tablets
(B) capsules
(C) syrups
(D) parenteral solutions
(E) topical lotions

279. With the rapid progress of legalized marijuana in the US, the pharmacist must be aware of the active chemical agents that are in marijuana. Which of the following are important components of marijuana?

I. IOP

II. CBD

III. THC

(A) I only (B) III only (C) I & II only
(D) II & III only (E) I, II, & III

280. Which of the following is/are used in the treatment of narcotic dependence?

I. Naltrexone

II. Methadone

III. Buprenorphine

(A) I only (B) III only (C) I & II only

(D) II & III only (E) I, II, & III

281. All of the following acronyms are related to prescription drug pricing EXCEPT

(A) DME (B) AWP (C) AAC

(D) EAC (E) MAC

282. Refusal of a patient to provide medical information for a patient prescription profile means that the pharmacist:

I. can fill the prescription at his/her discretion.

II. must call the patient's physician to confirm the patient's medical condition.

III. must tell the patient that the prescription may not be filled without the requested information.

(A) I only (B) III only (C) I & II only

(D) II & III only (E) I, II, & III

283. Which one of the following pieces of information is NOT encoded into a drug product's NDC?

(A) product's expiration date

(B) manufacturer

(C) package size

(D) drug name

(E) strength of a tablet

284. Federal guidelines require that the pharmacist should indicate the date on which a prescription refill is dispensed

(A) on the back of the paper prescription.

(B) on the front of the paper prescription.

(C) on the prescription label.

(D) in a special refill log book.

(E) on the counseling sheet given to the patient.

285. The body that is responsible for overseeing the selection of a nonproprietary name for a new drug is the:

(A) FDA (B) USAN (C) APhA

(D) USP/NF (E) FTC

286. Which of the following entities must be registered in order to participate in the prescribing or dispensing of isotretinoin?

I. prescribers

II. pharmacies

III. drug wholesalers

(A) I only (B) III only (C) I & II only

(D) II & III only (E) I, II, & III

287. The Electronic Orange Book uses the symbol "RLD", in a series of similar drug products to indicate:

(A) the drug products that have not been assessed

(B) that there is no bioequivalence problem

(C) the drug product that is preferred by most pharmacists for substitution

(D) the least expensive drug product

(E) the product used as a reference standard

288. The use of an FDA approved drug for a use that is not approved for the drug is best described as being:

(A) illegal (B) terminal (C) orphan

(D) off-label (E) unprofessional

289. Controlled substance prescriptions

I. may be written by typewriter (except for the prescriber's signature).

II. must have the name of the physician printed, stamped, typed, or hand-printed on it.

III. may be prepared by an agent of the prescriber for the prescriber's signature

(A) I only (B) III only (C) I & II only
(D) II & III only (E) I, II, & III

290. Oral authorization for additional refills on a schedule III prescription are acceptable as long as

I. the pharmacist gets a "cover" prescription from the prescriber within 7 days of the oral authorization.

II. the quantity of each additional refill authorized is not greater than the quantity authorized for the initial filling of the prescription.

III. the total quantity authorized does not exceed five refills within a six-month period from the date of issue of the original prescription.

(A) I only (B) III only (C) I & II only
(D) II & III only (E) I, II, & III

291. A physician shares with your pharmacy a topical moisturizing formula which contains a prescription drug. Which of the following would be appropriate actions for your pharmacy to take?

I. Fill prescriptions written by the physician for 120 grams of this formula.

II. Prepare a pound of the formula in anticipation of additional prescriptions or refills.

III. Prepare 50 x 120 g of the formula for sale from the physician's office.

(A) I only (B) III only (C) I & II only
(D) II & III only (E) I, II, & III

292. Which of the following is required to be on the labeling of the prescription container when the pharmacist fills a Schedule III controlled substance prescription?

I. Date of initial filling

II. Federal "Caution" warning

III. Number of dosage units dispensed

(A) I only (B) III only (C) I & II only

(D) II & III only (E) I, II, & III

293. A pharmacy chain with stores in several states must obtain

(A) a DEA number in each state that it owns a store.

(B) a DEA number for each individual pharmacy location.

(C) just one DEA number for the entire chain.

(D) a DEA number for each of the chain's regional offices.

(E) a DEA number for each Pharmacy Supervisor in the chain.

294. The requirement that pharmacists must offer to counsel patients concerning their prescriptions was included in which of the following congressional actions?

(A) Durham-Humphrey Amendment of 1951

(B) FD & C Act of 1938

(C) Omnibus Reconciliation Act of 1990

(D) Prescription Drug Marketing Act of 1987

(E) Kefauver-Harris Amendment of 1962

295. When explaining the Medicare Plan D program to a married couple, the pharmacist should emphasize that which of the following applies to each individual?

I. the original annual deductible

II. the monthly premium

III. the "donut hole"

(A) I only (B) III only (C) I & II only

(D) II & III only (E) I, II, & III

296. A customer had a prescription originally filled on December 1, 2015 and at that time acknowledged receiving the pharmacy's notice of privacy rights under HIPAA. She also receives a refill dispensed on January 2, 2016. What is the earliest date that the pharmacy may discard the patient's acknowledgment?

(A) 12/1/2016 (B) 1/2/2016 (C) 12/1/2021
(D) 1/2/2020 (E) never

297. Which of the following are exempt from registration under the Controlled Substance Act?

I. A foreign-trained physician
II. A U.S. Public Health Service physician
III. A U.S. Army physician

(A) I only (B) III only (C) I & II only
(D) II & III only (E) I, II, & III

298. Percogesic is an example of a product that is

(A) in Schedule II
(B) in Schedule III
(C) in Schedule IV
(D) in Schedule V
(E) not a controlled substance

299. Labels of commercial drug products that are intended for electrolyte replacement must state the concentration expressed in terms of:

I. weight or concentration
II. milliequivalents
III. millimoles

(A) I only (B) III only (C) I & II only
(D) II & III only (E) I, II, & III

300. Zolpidem is regulated by federal law in the same way as

(A) oxycodone

(B) buprenorphine

(C) phenobarbital

(D) lorazepam

(E) diphenoxylate/atropine combination

Answers to Sample Questions

1. C	25. A	49. A	73. A	97. C
2. C	26. B	50. E	74. A	98. E
3. B	27. A	51. D	75. A	99. C
4. A	28. B	52. B	76. C	100. A
5. E	29. C	53. B	77. E	101. B
6. D	30. B	54. C	78. B	102. E
7. A	31. D	55. D	79. B	103. D
8. E	32. D	56. A	80. A	104. E
9. A	33. A	57. B	81. C	105. E
10. C	34. E	58. D	82. B	106. C
11. D	35. B	59. A	83. E	107. D
12. D	36. D	60. E	84. D	108. E
13. E	37. D	61. E	85. A	109. D
14. E	38. B	62. B	86. B	110. A
15. B	39. C	63. A	87. C	111. E
16. A	40. A	64. D	88. E	112. A
17. B	41. B	65. A	89. D	113. A
18. A	42. D	66. D	90. C	114. B
19. B	43. E	67. C	91. E	115. C
20. E	44. D	68. E	92. D	116. B
21. D	45. C	69. D	93. E	117. B
22. E	46. A	70. B	94. A	118. A
23. C	47. C	71. E	95. D	119. C
24. B	48. B	72. B	96. D	120. D

121. B	147. B	174. D	200. B	226. C
122. C	148. D	175. C	201. A	227. E
123. E	149. B	176. A	202. D	228. A
124. A	150. B	177. D	203. E	229. B
125. E	151. A	178. E	204. C	230. A
126. D	152. D	179. E	205. B	231. C
127. C	153. A	180. D	206. D	232. E
128. C	154. B	181. E	207. D	233. B
129. E	155. A	182. B	208. C	234. E
130. D	156. D	183. C	209. B	235. A
131. C	157. B	184. C	210. C	236. B
132. A	158. E	185. E	211. E	237. D
133 C	159. A	186. B	212. E	238. D
134. D	160. C	187. B	213. D	239. A
135. E	162. D	188. C	214. B	240. E
136. E	163. A	189. C	215. C	241. B
137. D	164. C	190. D	216. A	242. E
138. C	165. B	191. D	217. E	243. E
139. A	166. C	192. A	218. D	244. E
140. D	167. D	193. A	219. A	245. A
141. E	168. D	194. D	220. A	246. E
142. C	169. C	195. B	221. D	247. E
143. C	170. A	196. C	222. D	248. A
144. C	171. B	197. E	223. E	249. C
145. E	172. B	198. C	224. D	250. C
146. A	173. D	199. E	225. A	251. E

252. E	263. D	274. E	285. B	296. C
253. B	264. C	275. B	286. E	297. D
254. A	265. A	276. B	287. E	298. E
255. C	266. C	277. E	288. D	299. D
256. E	267. C	278. D	289. E	300. D
257. A	268. B	279. D	290. D	
258. C	269. E	280. E	291. C	
259. B	270. B	281. A	292. C	
260. C	271. A	282. A	293. B	
261. A	272. D	283. A	294. C	
262. C	273. A	284. A	295. E	

Index

A

B

C

D

E

F

Q

R

S

T

U

V

W

X